Aromas of Wellness

Harnessing Nature's Essence for Health and Harmony

Casey Bright

Table of Contents

INTRODUCTION

Welcome to "Aromas of Wellness: Harnessing the Essence of Nature for Health and Harmony" In this book, we embark on a journey into the captivating world of aromatherapy and explore the profound healing potential of essential oils and aromatic compounds for holistic wellness. We will delve into the rich knowledge of aromatherapy and discover how the aromatic essences of plants can nourish our body, mind and soul and lead us to greater balance, vitality and harmony in our lives.

Across nations and civilizations, aromatherapy—the art and science of employing aromatic plant extracts to promote health and well-being—has been used for centuries. Aromatic herbs have long been valued for their medicinal qualities and spiritual significance, making them strong friends in the pursuit of enlightenment, healing, and transformation from ancient Egypt and China to Greece and India. We pay tribute to this age-old custom in "Aromas of Wellness," delving into its significance and practical applications in the contemporary era.

At the heart of aromatherapy is the belief in the interconnectedness of all living beings and the natural world. Essential oils, the primary tools of aromatherapy, are distilled from various parts of aromatic plants, including flowers, leaves, bark and roots, to capture the essence of the plant and its healing properties. Every essential oil has a distinct blend of bioactive substances that work in concert with our bodies to affect moods, energy levels, and physiological functions. By harnessing the power of these natural essences, we can support our body's innate healing abilities and cultivate a deeper sense of well-being.

In this book, we will explore the science, history, and practical applications of aromatherapy, giving you the knowledge and tools to incorporate this ancient healing art into your daily life. You will learn about the therapeutic properties of different essential oils and how to create customized blends and rituals. You will discover how you can use nature's aromatic essences to improve your health, vitality, and happiness. Whether you want to reduce stress, support your sleep or seek a moment of relaxation and rejuvenation, "Aromas of Wellness" offers guidance and inspiration on your path to more excellent health and harmony.

CHAPTER I

Foundations of Aromatherapy

Origins and History of Aromatherapy

The origins and history of aromatherapy are dated back thousands of years They are deeply woven into the fabric of human civilization and cultural practices. Aromatherapy has a long and varied history that spans continents and cultures and includes a wide range of customs, beliefs, and practices. It is the art and science of employing fragrant plant extracts for therapeutic reasons.

Egyptian, Mesopotamian, and Chinese medicine records trace back to a time when fragrant plants were used for medical purposes. Aromatic oils and resins were employed in embalming, medical preparations, and religious ceremonies in ancient Egypt. Fragrant materials with medicinal, purifying, and spiritual qualities, such cedarwood, frankincense, and myrrh, were highly prized. They were frequently used in embalming, which preserved the deceased's body. Herbal remedies and preventive properties were also attributed to aromatic herbs like juniper, rosemary, and thyme. They were used in medicinal preparations to treat various ailments and promote health and well-being.

In ancient China, aromatic plants and herbal medicines were central to traditional healing practices such as Traditional Chinese Medicine (TCM). Aromatic herbs and essential oils for medicinal purposes go back thousands of years. References to aromatic substances can be found in arcaic Chinese medical texts such as the Huangdi

Neijing (Inner Canon of the Yellow Emperor). Aromatic herbs such as ginger, cinnamon, and ginseng were prized for their ability to harmonize body, mind, and spirit. They treated various ailments, from indigestion to respiratory infections.

Aromatic herbs were prized for their therapeutic and medicinal qualities in classical Greece and Rome, where they were utilized to make ointments, perfumes, and infusions. The Greek physician Hippocrates, often called the "father of medicine," advocated aromatic herbs and essential oils for their healing properties and incorporated them into his medical treatments. Galen, a Roman physician, also wrote a great deal on the therapeutic uses of aromatic herbs and suggested using them to cure a range of conditions, from mental sickness to digestive issues.

Aromatherapy was very popular in Europe during the Middle Ages, but it was mostly utilized in religious and spiritual situations. Aromatic herbs and essential oils were used in religious ceremonies, rituals, and rites of passage because it was believed that they had healing, purifying, and protective properties. Monks and herbalists preserved and expanded the knowledge of aromatherapy by documenting the medicinal properties of aromatic plants and developing herbal remedies and preparations for various ailments.

During the Renaissance, interest in aromatherapy and herbal medicine revived as scholars and scientists rediscovered the wisdom of ancient civilizations and attempted to combine it with modern medical knowledge. Doctors such as Paracelsus and Nicholas Culpeper explored the therapeutic properties of aromatic plants and essential oils and incorporated them into their medical treatments. In addition, the invention of printing enabled the widespread dissemination of knowledge about aromatherapy and herbal medicine and led to the publication of numerous books and treatises on the subject.

In the 20th century, aromatherapy experienced a revival thanks to the pioneering work of personalities such as Rene-Maurice Gattefosse, a French drugstore who coined the term "aromatherapy" in the 1920s. Gattefosse came across the healing properties of lavender essential oil after he burned his hand in a laboratory accident and found that the oil promoted wound healing and scarring. He researched and promoted essential oils for medicinal purposes, laying the foundations for modern aromatherapy.

There was another key figure in the development of modern aromatherapy. She was Marguerite Maury, a French biochemist, and aromatherapist who pioneered the use of essential oils in massage and skin care. Maury was convinced that essential oils could penetrate the skin and influence the physiology of the body. It could also developed unique massage techniques and formulations for the treatment of various health conditions. Her work helped popularize aromatherapy as a holistic healing modality and paved the way for its integration into mainstream health practices.

In the second half of the 20th century and into the 21st century, aromatherapy had evolved. It was recognized worldwide as a complementary therapy in healthcare and wellness practices. Exploring the therapeutic properties of essential oils has increased, with studies investigating their effects on physical, emotional, and mental health. Aromatherapy has also become more accessible to the general public, with a wide range of products and tools available for home use, including essential oils, diffusers, massage oils and skincare products.

Today, aromatherapy is practiced and appreciated by millions of people around the world who use aromatic plants and essential oils for their healing, rejuvenating and restorative properties. From massage therapists and naturopaths to medical professionals and spa therapists, aromatherapy is used in a vast variety of settings to promote health, well-being, and relaxation. As attraction to natural and holistic approaches to health continues to grow, aromatherapy is likely to remain a valued and integral part of humanity's healing journey for generations to come.

The Science Behind Aromatherapy

Aromatherapy is often considered as an ancient art. It is increasingly supported by modern scientific research, revealing the intricate mechanisms essential oils exert in their therapeutic effects on the body and mind. This convergence of traditional wisdom and modern science has led to a deeper understanding of the science behind aromatherapy and shed light on the biochemical, physiological and psychological processes that underlie its effectiveness. This section explores the fascinating science behind aromatherapy and examines the fundamental principles, mechanisms of action and evidence-based applications that contribute to its growing recognition as a legitimate complementary therapy in modern healthcare.

Aromatherapy centers on essential oils and highly concentrated plant extracts that contain complex blends of bioactive compounds with diverse therapeutic properties. These compounds, including terpenes, phenols and esters, interact with the body in various ways, influencing physiological processes, neurotransmitter activity and cellular signaling pathways. One of the most important mechanisms by which essential oils exert their effect is through smell, i.e. the sense of smell. When inhaled, the volatile aromatic compounds in essential oils stimulate the olfactory receptors in the nasal cavity, triggering neuronal signals that are transmitted to the brain's limbic system, the seat of emotions, memory and autonomic functions. This oilfactory pathway establishes a direct link between the sense of smell and the limbic system, allowing essential oils to profoundly influence mood, perception and behavior.

On top of it, essential oils have pharmacological properties that were used to effectively treat various health conditions. The vast majoroty of essential oils have antimicrobial, anti-inflammatory, analgesic and antioxidant properties, which make them valuable agents for supporting immune function, relieving pain and inflammation, and protecting against oxidative stress and cellular damage. Tea tree oil, for example, is known for its antimicrobial properties and has been shown to interfere with the growth of bacteria, fungi and viruses, making it a popular treatment for skin infections, acne and respiratory conditions. Similarly, lavender oil, valued for its calming and soothing effects, has been found to modulate neurotransmitter activity and promote relaxation, making it a valuable remedy for stress, anxiety and sleep disorders.

In addition, research into the physiological effects of aromatherapy has shown that it affects the autonomic nervous system, the body's regulatory system that controls spontaneous functions such as heart rate, blood pressure and digestion. Researches have shown that inhaling certain essential oils can influence autonomic function, leading to changes in heart rate variability, blood pressure and respiratory rate. For example, inhaling lavender oil has been found to reduce sympathetic nervous system activity and increase parasympathetic nervous system activity, leading to a state of relaxation and calmness. Similarly, peppermint oil has been shown to improve cognitive performance and alertness by stimulating the central nervous system and increasing brain activity.

In addition, aromatherapy has been shown to have immunomodulatory effects by influencing immune cell activity and strengthening the body's defense mechanisms against pathogens and foreign invaders. Essential oils such as eucalyptus, oregano and thyme have been illustrated to stimulate immune cell activity, increase the production of cytokines and antibodies and improve the body's ability to fight infection. These immune-boosting effects make essential oils a valuable addition to the conventional treatment of respiratory infections, influenza and other infectious diseases.

In addition, new research suggests that aromatherapy may also have neuroprotective effects that could benefit brain health and cognitive function. Studies have shown that certain essential oils such as rosemary, lemon and frankincense contain bioactive blends that may preserve against neurodegenerative diseases such as Alzheimer's and Parkinson's by reducing oxidative stress, inflammation and neuronal damage. These neuroprotective effects can be marked the antioxidant, anti-inflammatory and anti-amyloid properties of the essential oils, which help to preserve neuronal function and prevent the accumulation of pathological proteins in the brain.

In addition, aromatherapy has been shown to have psychophysiological effects that affect mood, emotions and psychological well-being. Gasping essential oils can stimulate the release of neurotransmitters such as serotonin, dopamine and endorphins, which show a crucial role in regulating mood, pleasure and stress responses. For example, inhaling citrus oils such as bergamot and orange has been found to elevate mood and cut down symptoms of depression and anxiety, while inhaling floral oils such as rose and jasmine can induce feelings of calm and emotional balance. Moreover, studies have demonstrated that aromatherapy massage, a common use of essential oils, can lessen tension, elevate mood, and encourage relaxation by fusing the senses of touch and smell.

In a nutshell, the science behind aromatherapy provides compelling evidence of its therapeutic efficacy and physiological effects on the body and mind. From influencing the nervous system and immune function to the effects on mood, emotions and cognitive performance, aromatherapy offers a versatile approach to promoting health, well-being and vitality. As research progresses, our understanding of the science behind aromatherapy will continue to deepen, further cementing its role as a valuable complementary therapy in modern healthcare.

Essential Oils: Nature's Gift to Wellness

Essential oils, often referred to as nature's gift for well-being, have captivated mankind for centuries with their aromatic appeal and therapeutic properties. Essential oils are infused from various parts of aromatic plants, including flowers, leaves, bark and roots. They are highly concentrated extracts that contain a complex array of bioactive compounds with multiple medicinal and therapeutic benefits. From ancient civilizations to modern wellness practices, essential oils are revered for promoting physical, emotional and spiritual well-being. They endevour a holistic approach to health that is in harmony with the interconnectedness of nature and the human body.

The distinguishing characteristic of essential oils is their aromatic profile, which is created by volatile organic compounds that evaporate quickly at room temperature. These volatile compounds, including terpenes, phenols, aldehydes and esters, give each essential oil a distinctive fragrance and therapeutic properties. The fresh, citrusy aroma of lemon oil, for example, is due to the high concentration of limonene, a terpene known for its uplifting and mood-enhancing effects. The warm, woody scent of sandalwood oil, on the other hand, is due to its high content of santalol, a compound valued for its grounding and calming properties.

In addition, essential oils have numerous therapeutic properties that make them valuable allies in promoting health and well-being. Many essential oils have antimicrobial, anti-inflammatory, analgesic and antioxidant properties, making them effective agents for supporting immune function, relieving pain and inflammation and protecting against oxidative stress and cell damage. Tea tree oil, for example, is known for its antimicrobial properties and has been shown to supress the growth of bacteria, fungi and viruses, making it a popular treatment for skin infections, acne and respiratory conditions. Lavender oil, valued for its calming and soothing effects, has been shown to modulate neurotransmitter activity and promote relaxation, making it a valuable remedy for stress, anxiety and sleep disorders.

As well as, essential oils can be used in a vast majority of ways to promote health and well-being, including inhalation, topical application and internal use. Inhalation of essential oils is one of the most common methods of aromatherapy as it allows direct absorption of aromatic compounds into the bloodstream via the lungs. By inhaling essential oils, the volatile compounds are transported to the olfactory receptors in the nasal cavity, where they stimulate neuronal signals that are transmitted to the brain's limbic system, the seat of emotions, memory and autonomic functions. This olfactory pathway establishes a direct connection between the sense of smell and the brain, allowing essential oils to profoundly influence mood, perception and behavior.

In addition, topical application of essential oils is another popular method of aromatherapy as it allows for the direct absorption of bioactive compounds through the skin. When administered to the skin, the essential oils penetrate the epidermis and dermis, are absorbed into the bloodstream and distributed throughout the body. The topical applying of essential oils can be through massage, compresses, baths or skin care products so that the therapeutic agents can be targeted to specific areas of the body. Peppermint oil, for example, which is known for its cooling and pain-relieving properties, can be used topically to soothe sore muscles, relieve headaches and relieve tension.

On top of it, the internal use of essential oils is a less common but potentially effective method of aromatherapy when done properly and under the guidance of a qualified practitioner. Some essential oils are safe for intake internal use when properly diluted and taken in small doses, while others are best used externally or by inhalation. Essential oils can be used internally by adding them to food and drink, taking them in capsule form or using them as a dietary supplement. Lemon oil, for example, can be added to water as a refreshing and detoxifying drink. In contrast, oregano oil can be taken in capsule form to support immune function and digestive health.

What is more, essential oils may be used to create personal blends and formulations tailored to individual needs and preferences. By combining different essential oils in specific ratios, synergistic effects can be achieved, enhancing the therapeutic benefits of each oil and creating unique aroma profiles. For example, lavender, chamomile and bergamot oils may promote relaxation and reduce stress. In contrast, a blend of eucalyptus, peppermint and tea tree oils may support respiratory health and relieve congestion. In addition, essential oils can be combined with carrier oils, hydrosols and other natural ingredients to design a wide range of skin, hair and body care products that provide holistic solutions for beauty and self-care.

In summary, essential oils are nature's gift to wellbeing. They provide a holistic approach to health and wellbeing that takes into account all facets of human existence—physical, emotional, and spiritual. With their aromatic appeal and therapeutic properties, essential oils can uplift the spirit, soothe the body and rejuvenate the mind, offering a natural and sustainable alternative to conventional treatments. Whether inhaled, applied topically or taken internally, essential oils are a versatile and effective means of promoting health, harmony and vitality for individuals and communities worldwide.

CHAPTER II

The Impact of Aromas on Well-being

Exploring the Mind-Body Connection of aromatherapy

When exploring the mind-body connection of aromatherapy it unveils a profound interplay between our mental and physical well-being. Aromatherapy is showcasing how scent can influence our emotions, thoughts, and bodily functions. As the ancient practice of using aromatic plant can be extracted for therapeutic purposes, taps into this intricate relationship, harnessing the power of scent to promote holistic healing and balance. In this section, we delve into the fascinating world of the mind-body connection in aromatherapy, exploring the mechanisms, effects, and applications of scent on our mental and physical states.

At the heart of the mind-body connection in aromatherapy lies the olfactory system, a complex network of sensory receptors in the nasal cavity responsible for our sense of smell. When we inhale aromatic compounds from essential oils, they interact with olfactory receptors, triggering neural signals transmitted to the brain's limbic system, the seat of emotions, memory, and autonomic functions. This direct pathway between the sense of smell and the limbic system allows essential oils to profoundly affect our mood, cognition, and behavior. It can even influence on how we feel and perceive the world.

Moreover, research has shown that scent can evoke robust emotional responses and memories, often eliciting feelings of nostalgia, comfort, or relaxation. This phenomenon, known as the Proustian effect, highlights the deep connection between scent, memory, and emotion. It also suggest that certain aromas can transport us back in time and evoke vivid memories from our past. For example, the smell of lavender may remind us of a peaceful childhood garden, while the aroma of citrus may evoke memories of summer vacations by the beach. By leveraging the Proustian effect, aromatherapy can help us access and process buried emotions, memories, and traumas, offering a path to healing and self-discovery.

Furthermore, the mind-body connection in aromatherapy extends beyond emotions and memories to encompass physiological responses and bodily functions. Surveys have shown that inhaling certain essential oils can influence autonomic nervous system activity, leading to heart rate, blood pressure, and respiratory rate changes. For example, inhaling lavender oil has been found to reduce sympathetic nervous system activity and increase parasympathetic nervous system activity, resulting in a state of relaxation and calmness. Similarly, inhaling peppermint oil has been shown to enhance cognitive performance and alertness by stimulating the central nervous system and increasing brain activity.

In addition, scent can also impact our perception of pain and discomfort, with certain aromas having analgesic and pain-relieving properties. Research has shown that inhaling essential oils such as lavender, chamomile, and eucalyptus can reduce pain perception and alleviate symptoms of headaches, migraines, and muscle soreness. These analgesic effects are believed to be mediated through the reliefe of endorphins, our body's natural painkillers, and the modulation of neurotransmitter activity in the brain. By integrating aromatherapy into pain management protocols, individuals may experience relief from pain and discomfort without relying solely on pharmaceutical interventions.

Over and above, the mind-body connection in aromatherapy can also influence our immune function and overall health. Researches have shown that inhaling certain essential oils can stimulate immune cell activity, increase the production of cytokines and antibodies, and enhance the body's ability to fight infections. For example, with its potent antimicrobial properties, eucalyptus oil has been shown to inhibit the growth of bacteria, fungi, and viruses, making it a valuable ally in supporting respiratory health and immune function. By strengthening the body's natural defense mechanisms, aromatherapy can help counter illness and promote overall well-being.

Additionally, the mind-body connection in aromatherapy can play a role in supporting mental health and emotional well-being. Research has shown that inhaling essential oils such as lavender, bergamot, and frankincense can reduce indication of stress, anxiety, and depression, stimulating a sense of calmness, relaxation, and emotional balance. These mood-enhancing effects are believed to be mediated through the modulation of neurotransmitter activity in the brain, including the release of serotonin, dopamine, and gamma-aminobutyric acid (GABA), which show critical roles in regulating mood, pleasure, and stress response.

In conclusion, exploring the mind-body connection of aromatherapy reveals the profound influence of scent on our mental and physical well-being, highlighting the interconnectedness of our emotions, thoughts, and bodily functions. By harnessing the power of scent, aromatherapy sufggest a holistic way to health and wellness that addresses the root causes of imbalance and promotes harmony between mind, body, and spirit. Whether used to reduce stress, alleviate pain, or enhance immune function, aromatherapy promotes health, vitality, and resilience for individuals and communities alike.

How Aromatherapy Influences Emotions and Mood

Aromatherapy's influence on emotions and mood is a captivating aspect of its therapeutic potential, demonstrating the profound connection between scent and our psychological well-being. By inhaling aromatic compounds found in essential oils, aromatherapy provide a natural and holistic approach to managing emotions, promoting relaxation, and enhancing mood. In this section, we explore the mechanisms, effects, and applications of how aromatherapy influences emotions and mood, shedding light on its transformative power in promoting emotional well-being.

The olfactory system, responsible for our sense of smell, plays a central role in how aromatherapy influences emotions and mood. When we inhale the aromatic compounds from essential oils, they interact with olfactory receptors in the nasal cavity, triggering neural signals transmitted to the brain's limbic system. The limbic system, often referred to as the brain's emotional center, is responsible for processing emotions, memories, and behaviors. Essential oils can evoke robust emotional responses and influence our mood states by directly stimulating the limbic system.

Moreover, research has shown that certain aromatic compounds found in essential oils can modulate neurotransmitter activity in the brain, leading to mood and emotional well-being changes. For example, inhaling citrus oils such as bergamot, lemon, and orange has been found to uplift mood and smooth symptoms of depression and anxiety. This mood-enhancing effect is believed to be mediated through the relief of neurotransmitters such as serotonin and dopamine, which are critical in regulating mood, pleasure, and stress responses. Similarly, inhaling floral oils such as lavender rose and jasmine has been shown to promote relaxation and reduce stress and tension, creating a sense of calmness and emotional balance.

Furthermore, the therapeutic effects of aromatherapy on emotions and mood extend beyond the immediate sensory experience to encompass long-term benefits for emotional well-being. Regular use of aromatherapy can help to regulate mood, scale down feelings of anxiety and depression, and promote overall emotional resilience. By incorporating aromatherapy into daily self-care rituals, individuals can cultivate a more thorough sense of emotional awareness and balance, enhancing their capacity to cope with life's challenges and stressors.

Additionally, aromatherapy can be used as a powerful tool for managing specific emotional issues and mental health conditions. For instance, essential oils like lavender, chamomile, and sandalwood are commonly used to promote relaxation and alleviate symptoms of insomnia and sleep disorders. Before going to bed, these relaxing oils can be applied to a warm bath or diffused throughout the bedroom to build a peaceful atmosphere that encourages sound sleep. Similarly, essential oils such as bergamot, clary sage, and ylang-ylang are known for their mood-stabilizing and antidepressant properties, making them valuable allies in managing symptoms of depression and mood disorders.

Moreover, aromatherapy can be personalized to suit individual preferences and needs, allowing for tailored approaches to promoting emotional well-being. By blending different essential oils in specific ratios, synergistic effects can be achieved, enhancing the therapeutic benefits of each oil and creating unique aromatic profiles. For example, a blend of citrus oils such as bergamot, lemon, and grapefruit may uplift mood and increase energy levels. In contrast, a blend of floral oils such as rose, geranium, and neroli may soothe anxiety and promote emotional balance.

Furthermore, the ritualistic nature of aromatherapy can also contribute to its emotional and mood-enhancing effects. Creating a sacred space for aromatherapy rituals, such as diffusing essential oils, lighting candles, and playing soothing music, may signal to the brain that it is time to relax and unwind. By inplementing mindfulness practices such as deep breathing, meditation, and visualization into aromatherapy sessions, some people can submarine their connection to the present moment and enhance their emotional awareness and resilience.

In conclusion, aromatherapy's influence on emotions and mood suggest a holistic approach to promoting emotional well-being, enhancing mood, and fostering emotional resilience. By inhaling aromatic compounds found in essential oils. Aromatherapy can stimulate the limbic system, regulates neurotransmitter activity, and promotes relaxation, creating a profound sensory experience that uplifts the spirit and soothes the soul. Whether used to reduce stress, alleviate anxiety, or encourage relaxation, aromatherapy offers a natural and effective means of enhancing emotional well-being and fostering a deeper connection to oneself and others.

Aromatherapy and Physical Health

Aromatherapy, often recognized for its calming and mood-enhancing benefits, also holds significant promise for promoting physical health and well-being. Aromatherapy, which has its roots in the use of natural plant extracts called essential oils, provides a comprehensive method of treating a range of physical illnesses, from musculoskeletal pain to respiratory disorders. In this section, we explore how aromatherapy influences physical health, its mechanisms of action, evidence-based applications, and potential benefits for individuals seeking natural alternatives to conventional medical treatments.

One of the primary mechanisms through which aromatherapy influences physical health is the inhalation of aromatic compounds found in essential oils. When inhaled, these volatile compounds interact with olfactory receptors in the nasal cavity, triggering neural signals transmitted to the brain. From there, these signals can exert various physiological effects on the body, including heart rate, blood pressure, and respiratory rate changes. For example, inhaling essential oils such as eucalyptus, peppermint, and tea tree has been shown to have decongestant and expectorant properties, helping to relieve symptoms of respiratory congestion, cough, and sinusitis.

Moreover, aromatherapy can also impact physical health through its effects on the immune system. Many essential oils possess antimicrobial, antiviral, and immunomodulatory properties, making them valuable allies in supporting immune function and fighting infections. For example, tea tree oil, renowned for its antimicrobial properties, has been shown to inhibit the growth of bacteria, fungi, and viruses, making it an effective natural remedy for treating skin infections, wounds, and respiratory infections. Similarly, essential oils such as lavender, thyme, and oregano have been found to stimulate immune cell activity and enhance the body's ability to ward off pathogens and foreign invaders.

Furthermore, aromatherapy can alleviate pain and discomfort associated with various physical conditions. Many essential oils exhibit analgesic, anti-inflammatory, and muscle-relaxing properties, effectively reducing pain and promoting relaxation. For instance, essential oils like lavender, chamomile, and clary sage commonly alleviate headaches, migraines, and muscle tension symptoms. These calming oils can be applied topically through massage or added to bathwater to create a soothing and therapeutic experience.

Additionally, aromatherapy can play a role in promoting digestive health and gastrointestinal function. Specific essential oils, such as peppermint, ginger, and fennel, have been shown to have carminative and digestive-stimulating properties, helping to alleviate symptoms of indigestion, bloating, and nausea. These digestive oils can be ingested in small doses, added to herbal teas, or applied topically to the abdomen to support digestive comfort and overall well-being.

Moreover, aromatherapy can also have cardiovascular benefits, including scaling down heart rate, blood pressure, and cholesterol levels. Essential oils: lavender, ylang-ylang, and bergamot have been found to have vasodilatory and hypotensive effects, helping to promote relaxation and improve circulation. By incorporating aromatherapy into daily self-care routines, individuals can experience cardiovascular benefits such as reduced stress, improved sleep, and enhanced overall heart health.

Furthermore, aromatherapy can support hormonal balance and reproductive health, offering natural solutions for menstrual cramps, menopausal symptoms, and hormonal imbalances. Oils such as clary sage, geranium, and rose are known for their hormone-balancing and uterine-regulating properties, making them valuable allies for women's health and well-being. These hormone-balancing oils can be applied topically to the abdomen or added to a warm bath to help alleviate symptoms of PMS, menstrual cramps, and menopausal discomfort.

Additionally, aromatherapy can be used as part of a far-reaching approach to managing chronic conditions such as arthritis, fibromyalgia, and chronic pain syndromes. Many essential oils possess anti-inflammatory, analgesic, and muscle-relaxing properties, making them effective agents for reducing pain and improving the quality of life for individuals with chronic pain. By incorporating aromatherapy into their daily self-care routines, some people can experience relief from pain and discomfort without relying solely on pharmaceutical interventions.

In summary, aromatherapy offers a holistic approach to promoting physical health and well-being, addressing various conditions and symptoms through inhalation, topical application, and internal use of essential oils. From respiratory congestion to digestive discomfort, from pain relief to immune support, aromatherapy offers natural and great solutions for individuals seeking to enhance their physical health and vitality. By harnessing the healing power of plants and incorporating aromatherapy into daily self-care routines, individuals can exposure the transformative benefits of this ancient practice for their physical, emotional, and spiritual well-being.

CHAPTER III

Essential Oils and Their Benefits

Benefit of Lavender: The Universal Oil for Relaxation

Lavender often hailed as the universal oil for relaxation is revered in aromatherapy for its myriad therapeutic benefits and soothing properties. Lavender essential oil is extracted from the blossoms of the Lavandula angustifolia plant and has been used for generations to improve general wellbeing, reduce stress, and encourage relaxation. In this section, we examine the many advantages of lavender oil, including its mechanisms of action, evidence-based uses, and capacity to foster calm and relaxation in people looking for all-natural ways to reduce stress and unwind.

One of the primary mechanisms through which lavender oil promotes relaxation is its ability to modulate neurotransmitter activity in the brain, particularly the neurotransmitter gamma-aminobutyric acid (GABA). GABA is an inhibitory neurotransmitter that aid regulate neuronal excitability and promote calmness and relaxation. Lavender oil consist of mixes such as linalool and linalyl acetate, which have been found to enhance GABA receptor activity and increase GABA levels in the brain. By modulating GABA neurotransmission, lavender oil helps induce relaxation and tranquility, making it an effecient remedy for reducing stress, anxiety, and tension.

Moreover, lavender oil has been found to have anxiolytic, or anxiety-reducing, effects on the central nervous system, making it a valuable ally in managing symptoms of anxiety and stress-related disorders. Studies has shown that inhaling lavender oil can help to reduce subjective feelings of fear, promote relaxation, and improve mood. For example, a research published in the Journal of Alternative and Complementary Medicine discoverd that inhaling lavender oil vapor for just 15 minutes significantly reduced anxiety levels in participants compared to a control group. These findings suggest that lavender oil has the potential to be used as a natural remedy for anxiety and stress management.

Furthermore, lavender oil has been found to have sedative properties, making it a practical aid for promoting relaxation and improving sleep quality. Research has shown that inhaling lavender oil or administer it topically to the skin can help enhance sleep quality, increase sleep duration, and reduce insomnia symptoms. For example, a survey appeared in the journal Data-Based Complementary and Alternative Medicine showed that inhaling lavender oil vapor before bedtime significantly improved sleep quality and reduced insomnia symptoms in participants with sleep disorders. These sedative effects are believed to be mediated through the modulation of neurotransmitter activity in the brain, including the release of serotonin, dopamine, and norepinephrine, which play critical roles in regulating sleep-wake cycles and promoting relaxation.

Additionally, lavender oil has been found to have analgesic or pain-relieving properties, making it an effective remedy for reducing pain and discomfort associated with various conditions. Research has shown that applying lavender oil topically to the skin can help alleviate headaches, migraines, and muscle tension symptoms. For example, a study published in the journal European Neurology discovered that inhaling lavender oil for 15 minutes fundamentaly reduced the severity of migraine headaches and improved symptoms in participants compared to a control group. These analgesic effects are believed to be mediated through the inhibition of pain signaling pathways in the brain and the modulation of neurotransmitter activity in the central nervous system.

Moreover, lavender oil has been found to be anti-inflammatory features making it a valuable ally in promoting skin health and reducing inflammation. Research has shown that applying lavender oil topically to the skin can help to soothe irritation, reduce redness, and promote wound healing. For example, a study published in the Evidence-Based Complementary and Alternative Medicine journal found that applying lavender oil to surgical wounds significantly reduced inflammation and promoted faster healing compared to a control group. These anti-inflammatory effects are believed to be mediated through inhibiting pro-inflammatory cytokines and modulating immune cell activity in the skin.

Furthermore, lavender oil has been found to have antioxidant features, making it a valuable ally in protecting against oxidative stress and cellular damage. Research has shown that inhaling lavender oil or adminestering it topically to the skin can help neutralize free radicals, reduce oxidative damage, and promote cellular repair. For example, a study published in the Phytomedicine Journal found that inhaling lavender oil vapor for 60 minutes significantly reduced oxidative stress markers in participants compared to a control group. These antioxidant effects are believed to be mediated through activating antioxidant enzymes and scavenging reactive oxygen species in the body.

In conclusion, lavender oil stands out as a universal oil for relaxation, offering a wide range of therapeutic benefits for promoting physical, emotional, and mental well-being. From reducing stress and anxiety to promoting relaxation and improving sleep quality, lavender oil offers natural and effective ways for individuals seeking to enhance their overall health and vitality. By harnessing the soothing properties of lavender oil through inhalation, topical application, or aromatherapy, individuals can go through the transformative benefits of this ancient remedy for relaxation and tranquility.

Peppermint: Energizing and Invigorating

Peppermint has its refreshing aroma and invigorating properties. It is known that peppermint stands out as a versatile essential oil renowned for energizing and revitalizing the mind and body. It was derived from the Mentha piperita plant, its essential oil has a long history of use in traditional medicine and aromatherapy for its myriad therapeutic benefits. In this section, we explore the diverse benefits of peppermint oil, examining its mechanisms of action, evidence-based applications, and potential for promoting energy, focus, and vitality in individuals seeking natural solutions for fatigue and lethargy.

One of the primary mechanisms through which peppermint oil promotes energy and invigoration is its ability to stimulate the central nervous system and increase alertness and mental clarity. Peppermint oil consist of compounds such as menthol and menthone, which have been found to have stimulating and uplifting effects on the brain. During inhalation or appliying topically to the skin, these compounds interact with olfactory receptors in the nasal cavity, triggering neural signals transmitted to the brain's limbic system and prefrontal cortex. From there, these signals can enhance cognitive function, increase attention, and promote feelings of wakefulness and alertness, making peppermint oil an effective remedy for combating fatigue and mental fog.

Moreover, peppermint oil has been found to have analgesic or pain-relieving properties, making it a practical aid for reducing physical discomfort and promoting mobility and flexibility. Research has shown that applying peppermint oil topically to the skin can help alleviate muscle soreness, tension headaches, and joint pain symptoms. For example, a study published in the Journal of Clinical Nursing found that applying peppermint oil to the temples significantly reduced the severity and duration of tension headaches in participants compared to a placebo. These analgesic effects are believed to be mediated through the inhibition of pain signaling pathways in the brain and the modulation of neurotransmitter activity in the central nervous system.

Furthermore, peppermint oil has been found to be anti-inflammatory properties, securing it a valuable ally in promoting musculoskeletal health and reducing inflammation. Research has shown that applying peppermint oil topically to the skin can help to soothe inflammation, reduce swelling, and promote tissue repair.

For example, a study which was put out in journal "the European Journal of Physical and Rehabilitation Medicine" showed that applying peppermint oil to the skin significantly reduced inflammation and pain in patients with fibromyalgia compared to a placebo. These anti-inflammatory effects are believed to be mediated through inhibiting pro-inflammatory cytokines and modulating immune cell activity in the affected tissues.

Additionally, peppermint oil has been found to have antimicrobial features, making it an effective remedy for promoting oral health and combating oral infections. Research has shown that peppermint oil exhibits broad-spectrum antimicrobial activity against bacteria, fungi, and viruses, effectively inhibiting the growth of oral pathogens and reducing the risk of dental infections. For example, a study published in the Journal of International Oral Health found that mouthwash containing peppermint oil significantly reduced plaque accumulation and gingivitis in participants compared to a placebo. These antimicrobial effects are believed to be mediated through disrupting microbial cell membranes and inhibiting microbial enzyme activity.

Moreover, peppermint oil has been found to have digestive-stimulating properties, making it a valuable ally in promoting gastrointestinal health and alleviating symptoms of indigestion, bloating, and nausea. Research has shown that inhaling peppermint oil or consuming peppermint tea can help to stimulate digestive enzymes, increase bile production, and improve gastrointestinal motility. For example, a study published in the journal Digestive Diseases and Sciences found that peppermint oil capsules significantly reduced symptoms of irritable bowel syndrome (IBS) in participants compared to a placebo. These digestive-stimulating effects are believed to be mediated through the relaxation of gastrointestinal smooth muscle, leading to improved digestion and reduced symptoms of gastrointestinal discomfort.

Furthermore, peppermint oil has been found to have cooling and soothing effect, making it an effective remedy for promoting skin health and relieving symptoms of sunburn, itching, and inflammation. Research has shown that applying peppermint oil topically to the skin can help to soothe irritation, reduce redness, and promote wound healing. For instance, a study published in the Journal of Cosmetic Science found that peppermint oil significantly reduced skin inflammation and advanced wound healing in animal models. These cooling and soothing effects are believed to be mediated through the activation of the skin's transient receptor potential (TRP) channels, leading to a sensation of coolness and relief.

In conclusion, peppermint oil offers many therapeutic benefits for promoting energy, invigoration, and vitality. From stimulating the central nervous system and increasing mental clarity to relieving physical discomfort and promoting musculoskeletal health, peppermint oil offers natural and effective keys for individuals seeking to enhance their overall well-being. By harnessing the energizing and invigorating properties of peppermint oil through inhalation, topical application, or aromatherapy, people can experience the transformative benefits of this versatile essential oil for promoting energy, focus, and vitality in their daily lives.

Tea Tree: Nature's Antibacterial Agent

Tea tree oil has a well-earned reputation as nature's antibacterial agent because it is made from the leaves of the Australian original Melaleuca alternifolia tree. Due to its strong antibacterial qualities, tea tree oil has been used medicinally by Indigenous Australians for centuries. In this section, we explore the diverse benefits of tea tree oil, examining its mechanisms of action, evidence-based applications, and potential for promoting antibacterial activity and overall health in individuals seeking natural solutions for skin care, oral health, and wound care.

One of the primary mechanisms through which tea tree oil exerts its antibacterial effects is its high concentration of terpenes, particularly terpinene-4-ol. Terpinen-4-ol is a potent antimicrobial compound that has been shown to inhibit the growth of bacteria, fungi, and viruses. Tea tree oil disrupts the cellular membranes and metabolic processes of microorganisms by penetrating their cell walls when applied topically to the skin or mucous membranes. As a result, tea tree oil effectively treats a variety of bacterial diseases by killing off microorganisms and preventing their growth and colonization.

Furthermore, it has been shown that tea tree oil possesses anti-inflammatory qualities, which makes it a useful tool for lowering inflammation and encouraging the healing of wounds. According to research, topically applying tea tree oil to the skin can aid in tissue repair, reduce redness, and soothe irritation. In the Journal of

Investigative Dermatology, for instance, a study indicated that, in animal models, tea tree oil greatly sped up wound healing and decreased inflammation. It is thought that these anti-inflammatory benefits are achieved via immune cell activity modulation in the afflicted tissues and pro-inflammatory cytokine inhibition.

Furthermore, it has been shown that tea tree oil possesses antifungal qualities, which enable it to effectively suppress the growth of fungus like Candida albicans, which is the culprit behind yeast infections. According to study, topical use of tea tree oil to the skin or mucous membranes may help lessen fungal infection symptoms like burning, itching, and discharge. For instance, a study that was published in the Journal of Antimicrobial Chemotherapy discovered that both in vitro and in vivo growth of Candida albicans was greatly inhibited by tea tree oil. It is thought that the rupture of fungal cell membranes and the suppression of fungal enzyme activity are the mechanisms by which these antifungal actions are mediated.

Furthermore, it has been shown that tea tree oil possesses antiviral qualities, which enable it to effectively impede the growth of viruses like herpes simplex virus (HSV), which is the culprit behind cold sores. According to research, topically applying tea tree oil to the skin helps hasten the healing of cold sores and lessen the frequency and intensity of herpes outbreaks. For instance, compared to a placebo, tea tree oil dramatically shortened the participants' cold sores' duration and intensity, according to a study published in the journal Phytotherapy Research. It is thought that these antiviral actions are achieved by immune cell activity regulation in the afflicted tissues and prevention of virus replication.

Moreover it has been shown that tea tree oil possesses antibacterial qualities, which enable it to effectively cleanse wounds and avert infection. Studies have demonstrated the benefits of topically administering tea tree oil to small wounds, scrapes, and abrasions in terms of wound cleansing, microbial reduction, and wound healing.Research has shown that incorporating tea tree oil into personal care products such as deodorants, foot powders, and mouthwashes can help to control body odor, foot odor, and bad breath. For example, a study published in the journal Oral Microbiology and Immunology found that mouthwash containing tea tree oil significantly reduced oral bacteria and malodor in participants compared to a placebo. These deodorizing effects are believed to be mediated by inhibiting microbial growth and neutralizing volatile organic compounds responsible for odor.

In conclusion, tea tree oil offers many therapeutic benefits for promoting antibacterial activity and overall health. From inhibiting the growth of bacteria, fungi, and viruses to reducing inflammation, promoting wound healing, and controlling body odor, tea tree oil offers natural and effective key for those who is seeking to enhance their skincare, oral health, and wound care routines. By harnessing the potent antimicrobial properties of tea tree oil through topical application, inhalation, or aromatherapy, people can experience the transformative benefits of this versatile essential oil for promoting health and well-being.

Eucalyptus: Respiratory Support and Clearing Congestion

Eucalyptus, renowned for its invigorating aroma and therapeutic properties, is a powerful essential oil widely celebrated for providing respiratory support and clearing congestion. Essential oil of eucalyptus, which comes from the leaves of the eucalyptus tree (especially, Eucalyptus globulus and Eucalyptus radiata), has been used for generations in traditional medicine, especially in

Aboriginal Australian tribes. In this section, we explore the diverse benefits of eucalyptus oil, examining its mechanisms of action, evidence-based applications, and potential for promoting respiratory health and wellness in individuals seeking natural solutions for respiratory diseases such as coughs, colds, and sinus congestion.

One of the primary mechanisms through which eucalyptus oil supports respiratory health is its ability to act as a natural expectorant and decongestant. Eucalyptus oil contains compounds such as cineole, also known as eucalyptol, which have been found to have mucolytic properties, meaning they help to clear up and thin mucus in the respiratory tract. Eucalyptus oil can help to relieve congestion, loosen mucus, and aid in the ejection of mucus from the lungs, bronchi, and nasal passages when applied topically or inhaled into the chest. This makes eucalyptus oil an effective remedy for relieving symptoms of respiratory congestion, including coughing, wheezing, and difficulty breathing.

Moreover, eucalyptus oil has been found to have bronchodilator properties, meaning it helps to relax and free the airways and making it easier to breathe. Research has shown that inhaling eucalyptus oil vapor can help dilate bronchial passages, increase airflow to the lungs, and improve respiratory function in individuals with such diseases as asthma, bronchitis, and chronic obstructive pulmonary disease (COPD). For example, a study published in the journal Respiratory Medicine found that inhaling eucalyptus oil vapor significantly improved lung function and reduced asthma symptoms in participants compared to a placebo. These bronchodilator effects are believed to be mediated through the relaxation of smooth muscle in the airway walls and the inhibition of inflammatory mediators that contribute to airway constriction.

Furthermore, eucalyptus oil has been found to be antimicrobial features, making it effective in inhibiting the raise of bacteria, viruses, and fungi that can contribute to respiratory infections. Research has shown that eucalyptus oil exhibits broad-spectrum antimicrobial activity against respiratory pathogens such as Streptococcus pneumoniae, Haemophilus influenzae, and influenza virus. For example, a study published in the journal BMC Immunology found that eucalyptus oil significantly inhibited the growth of respiratory pathogens in vitro and in vivo. These antimicrobial effects are believed to be mediated by disrupting microbial cell membranes and inhibiting microbial enzyme activity, making eucalyptus oil a valuable ally in preventing and treating respiratory infections.

Additionally, eucalyptus oil has been found to be anti-inflammatory which make it effective in reducing inflammation of the respiratory tract and alleviating symptoms of respiratory diseases like asthma, bronchitis, and sinusitis. Research has shown that eucalyptus oil contains compounds such as alpha-pinene and 1,8-cineole, that have been found to inhibit the production of inflammatory cytokines and reduce inflammation in the lungs and nasal passages. It was proved, in a study which was published in the journal Pulmonary Pharmacology & Therapeutics found that inhaling eucalyptus oil vapor significantly reduced airway inflammation and improved lung function in animal models of asthma. These anti-inflammatory effects make eucalyptus oil a valuable remedy for promoting respiratory health and alleviating symptoms of inflammatory respiratory conditions.

Moreover, eucalyptus oil has been found to be analgesic properties, making it efficient in reducing pain and discomfort associated with respiratory conditions such as sore throat, coughing, and chest congestion. Research has shown that eucalyptus oil contains compounds such as terpenoids and flavonoids, which have been found to have pain-relieving effects and prevent the conduct of pain signals in the nervous system. For example, a study which appeared in Evidence-Based Complementary and Alternative Medicine found that inhaling eucalyptus oil vapor significantly reduced throat pain and coughing in those who have problems with acute upper respiratory tract infections. These analgesic effects make eucalyptus oil a valuable remedy for promoting comfort and relieving symptoms of respiratory discomfort.

Taking everything into account, eucalyptus oil offers many therapeutic benefits for promoting respiratory support and clearing congestion. From acting as a natural expectorant and decongestant to dilating bronchial passages, inhibiting microbial growth, reducing inflammation, and relieving pain, eucalyptus oil offers natural and perfect solutions for individuals seeking to enhance their respiratory health and well-being. By harnessing the therapeutic properties of eucalyptus oil through inhalation, topical application, or aromatherapy, individuals can experience the transformative benefits of this versatile essential oil for promoting respiratory health, vitality, and overall wellness.

Rosemary: Mental Clarity and Focus

Rosemary is a fragrant herb with a long history of culinary and medicinal use, it is known for its ability to build up mental clarity and enhance focus. Extracted from the Rosmarinus officinalis plant leaves, rosemary essential oil has been used for centuries because it was known for its refreshing aroma and therapeutic properties. In this section, we delve into the diverse benefits of rosemary oil, exploring its mechanisms of action, evidence-based applications, and potential for enhancing cognitive function and mental well-being in individuals seeking natural solutions for concentration, memory, and mental fatigue.

One of the primary mechanisms through which rosemary oil promotes mental clarity, and focus is its ability to stimulate the central nervous system and increase alertness and cognitive function. Rosemary oil consist of parts such as 1,8-cineole, also known as eucalyptol, which have been found to have stimulating and neuroprotective effects on the brain. Being inhaled or applied topically to the skin, these compounds interact with olfactory receptors in the nasal cavity, triggering neural signals that are transmitted to the brain's limbic system and prefrontal cortex. From there, these signals can enhance cognitive function, increase attention, and promote feelings of wakefulness and alertness, making rosemary oil an effective remedy for combating mental fatigue and improving concentration.

Moreover, rosemary oil has been found to have memory-enhancing properties, making it effective in improving cognitive performance and supporting learning and retention. Research has shown that inhaling rosemary oil vapor or administered it topically to the skin can help enhance memory recall, increase information processing speed, and improve overall brain function. For example, a study published in the journal Therapeutic Advances in Psychopharmacology found that inhaling rosemary oil vapor significantly improved cognitive performance and mood in participants compared to a control group. These memory-enhancing effects are believed to be mediated through the modulation of neurotransmitter activity in the brain, including the release of acetylcholine, a neurotransmitter involved in learning and memory.

Furthermore, rosemary oil has been found to have antioxidant properties, making it effective in protecting against oxidative stress and cellular damage in the brain. Research has shown that rosemary oil consist of partickles such as rosmarinic acid and carnosic acid, which have been found to neutralize free radicals, reduce oxidative damage, and promote neuronal survival. For example, a study published in the journal Food Chemistry found that rosemary extract significantly raised antioxidant enzyme activity and also reduced oxidative stress markers in the brains of animal models. These antioxidant effects are believed to be mediated through activating antioxidant enzymes and the scavenging of reactive oxygen species in the brain, making rosemary oil a valuable ally in protecting against age-related cognitive decline and neurodegenerative diseases.

Additionally, rosemary oil has been found to have mood-enhancing properties, making it effective in reducing symptoms of stress, anxiety, and depression. Research has shown that inhaling or applying rosemary oil vapor topically to the skin can help develop relaxation, reduce cortisol levels, and improve mood. For example, a study published in the journal Complementary Therapies in Medicine found that inhaling rosemary oil vapor significantly reduced cortisol levels and subjective feelings of stress in participants undergoing a stress-inducing task. These mood-enhancing effects are believed to be mediated through the modulation of neurotransmitter activity in the brain which includes the release of serotonin and dopamine, neurotransmitters involved in regulating mood and emotions.

Moreover, rosemary oil has been found to have anti-inflammatory properties, making it effecient in reducing inflammation in the brain and promoting cognitive health. The study has shown that rosemary oil contains compounds such as carnosol and carnosic acid, which have been found to inhibit the production of inflammatory cytokines and reduce neuroinflammation. For example, a study published in the journal Neurochemistry International found that rosemary extracts significantly reduced neuroinflammation and oxidative stress in animal dummy of Alzheimer's disease. These anti-inflammatory effects are believed to be mediated through inhibiting pro-inflammatory signaling pathways and modulating immune cell activity in the brain.

On a final way, rosemary oil offers many therapeutic benefits for promoting mental clarity, focus, and cognitive function. From stimulating the central nervous system and enhancing memory to protecting against oxidative stress and reducing inflammation in the brain, rosemary oil offers natural and perfect solutions for individuals seeking to improve their cognitive health and mental well-being. By harnessing the cognitive-enhancing and mood-boosting properties of rosemary oil through inhalation, topical application, or aromatherapy, some people say that they can experience the transformative benefits of this versatile essential oil for promoting mental clarity, focus, and overall cognitive vitality.

Citrus Oils: Uplifting and Refreshing

Citrus oils which come from the peels of citrus fruits like oranges, lemons, limes, and grapefruits, are celebrated for their uplifting and refreshing aroma and numerous therapeutic benefits. These essential oils have been used for centuries in traditional medicine and aromatherapy to invigorate the senses, uplift the mood, and promote overall well-being. In this section, we explore the diverse benefits of citrus oils. We examine their mechanisms of action, evidence-based applications, and potential for enhancing mood, reducing stress, and promoting relaxation in individuals seeking natural solutions for emotional support and mental clarity.

One of the primary mechanisms through which citrus oils uplift and refresh the mind and body is their ability to stimulate the olfactory system and trigger neural signals that promote feelings of happiness and well-being. Citrus oils contain compounds such as limonene and linalool, which have been found to have mood-enhancing and stress-reducing effects. When inhaled or diffused into the air, these compounds interact with olfactory receptors in the nasal cavity, triggering the release of neurotransmitters such as serotonin and dopamine, that are related to feelings of pleasure and relaxation. This makes citrus oils an effective remedy for lifting the spirits, reducing anxiety and depression, and promoting a sense of calm and contentment.

Moreover, citrus oils have been found to have energizing and revitalizing properties, making them effective in combating fatigue and mental exhaustion. Research has shown that inhaling citrus oil vapors or excecuted them topically to the skin can help to increase alertness, improve concentration, and boost cognitive function. For example, a research that appeared in the journal Evidence-Based Complementary and Alternative Medicine located that inhaling lemon essential oil significantly increased alertness and improved cognitive performance in participants compared to a placebo. These energizing effects are believed to be mediated through the activation of neurotransmitter activity in the brain, including the release of norepinephrine and acetylcholine, neurotransmitters involved in arousal and attention.

Furthermore, citrus oils have been found to have antimicrobial properties, making them effective in purifying the air and disinfecting surfaces. Research has shown that citrus oils contain compounds such as citral and citronellal, which have been found to witholded the growth of bacteria, viruses, and fungi that can cause illness and infection. For example, a study published in the journal Letters in Applied Microbiology found that lemon essential oil significantly reduced the growth of bacteria such as Escherichia coli and Staphylococcus aureus in vitro. These antimicrobial effects make citrus oils a valuable ally in promoting a clean and healthy environment, particularly during illness or seasonal allergies.

Additionally, citrus oils have been found to have antioxidant properties, making them effective in protecting against oxidative stress and cellular damage. Research has shown that citrus oils contain features such as flavonoids and polyphenols, which have been found to neutralize free radicals, reduce inflammation, and promote cellular repair. For example, a study published in Food Chemistry found that orange essential oil significantly increased antioxidant enzyme activity and decreased oxidative stress markers in animal models. These antioxidant effects are believed to be mediated through activating antioxidant enzymes and scavenging reactive oxygen species, making citrus oils a valuable ally in promoting overall health and longevity.

Moreover, citrus oils have been found to have appetite-suppressing properties, making them effective in supporting weight management and promoting healthy eating habits. Research has shown that inhaling or diffusing citrus oil vapors into the air can help reduce cravings, increase satiety, and improve mood. For example, a study published in the journal Neurological Research found that inhaling grapefruit essential oil significantly reduced appetite and food intake in participants compared to a control group. These appetite-suppressing effects are believed to be mediated through the activation of neurotransmitter activity in the brain, which includes the release of serotonin and dopamine, neurotransmitters involved in regulating appetite and mood.

As can be seen, citrus oils offer many therapeutic benefits for promoting upliftment, refreshment, and overall well-being. From stimulating the senses and boosting mood to combating fatigue, purifying the air, and supporting weight management, citrus oils offer natural and effective solutions for individuals seeking to enhance their emotional support, mental clarity, and physical health. By harnessing the mood-enhancing and stress-reducing properties of citrus oils through inhalation, topical application, or aromatherapy, some individuals can experience the transformative benefits of these versatile essential oils for promoting happiness, relaxation, and vitality in their daily lives.

CHAPTER IV

Aromatherapy Techniques and Practices

Inhalation Technique: Harnessing the Power of Scent

Inhalation is a fundamental technique in aromatherapy, harnessing the power of scent to deliver therapeutic benefits to the mind and body. This method involves breathing in the aromatic molecules of essential oils, which then interact with the olfactory system and the brain, triggering a cascade of physiological and psychological responses. Through inhalation, essential oils can promote relaxation, reduce stress, alleviate respiratory symptoms, and enhance mood, making it a versatile and practical therapeutic approach for promoting holistic well-being.

One of the primary benefits of inhalation is its skill to promote relaxation and reduce stress. When inhaling essential oils, aromatic molecules travel through the nasal passages and stimulate olfactory receptors, which are directly connected to the limbic system in the brain—the area responsible for regulating emotions and stress responses. Aromatherapy oils, including lavender, chamomile, and bergamot, have been well researched for their ability to calm and reduce anxiety when inhaled. Inhaling these oils can be a very useful tool for stress management and mental well-being, as research has demonstrated that they can assist to lower heart rate, blood pressure, and increase sensations of relaxation and peace.

Besides, inhalation is a very powerful tool for supporting respiratory health and reducing symptoms related to the respiratory system. Because of their decongestant, expectorant, and antibacterial qualities, essential oils including eucalyptus, peppermint, and tea tree have long been used to enhance respiratory function. These oils have the ability to clear nasal passages, lessen airway inflammation, and stop the spreading of bacteria and viruses that can create a cause for respiratory infections when breathed. Research has shown that inhaling steam infused with essential oils can provide rapid relief from congestion, coughing, and sinusitis symptoms, making inhalation a preferred method for addressing respiratory issues.

Furthermore, inhalation is an effective way to enhance mood and promote mental clarity. Essential oils such as lemon, rosemary, and peppermint are renowned for their refreshing and uplifting properties when inhaled. These oils can help to increase alertness, improve concentration, and boost cognitive function, making them ideal for enhancing productivity and mental performance. Research has shown that inhaling these stimulating oils can help increase neurotransmitters such as serotonin and dopamine in the brain, which are linked to feelings of happiness, motivation, and focus. Through the integration of inhalation techniques into everyday routines, people can harness the power of fragrance to elevate their mood, boost their energy, and encourage mental clarity all day long.

By the same token, inhalation is a safe and convenient method for administering essential oils, making it accessible to people of all ages and health conditions. Unlike topical application or ingestion, inhalation does not require dilution or special preparation and can be easily incorporated into daily rituals such as aromatherapy diffusers, steam inhalation, or aromatic baths. This makes inhalation ideal for individuals seeking natural remedies for various health concerns, from stress relief and respiratory support to mood enhancement and cognitive function.

In conclusion, inhalation is a powerful technique for harnessing the therapeutic benefits of essential oils and promoting holistic well-being. When inhaled with the aromatic molecules of essential oils, individuals can experience myriad benefits, including relaxation, stress reduction, respiratory support, mood enhancement, and mental clarity. Whether through aromatherapy diffusers, steam inhalation, or aromatic baths, inhalation offers a convenient and effective way to implement essential oils into daily routines and promote health and vitality naturally. By exploring the diverse benefits of inhalation and integrating it into daily self-care practices, individuals can experience the transformative power of scent and enhance their overall well-being.

Topical Application: Massage and Skin Care

The topical application of essential oils, mainly through massage and skin care, offers many benefits for physical and emotional well-being. By dilution with carrier oil, essential oils are applied topically to the skin, facilitating absorption into the bloodstream and targeted medicinal effects. Topical application is a versatile and useful way to utilize the medicinal characteristics of essential oils, as it may be used to enhance overall health, relieve muscle tension, and promote relaxation.

The capacity of topical treatment to induce relaxation and release tense muscles through massage is one of its main advantages. Because of their relaxing and analgesic qualities, essential oils like lavender, chamomile, and peppermint have long been utilized in massage therapy. When diluted and applied to the skin, these oils penetrate the dermal layers and interact with receptors in the underlying tissues, triggering a cascade of physiological responses. Studies have indicated that applying essential oils during a massage might alleviate tenseness in the muscles, enhance suppleness, and foster calmness by inducing the release of endorphins, which are the body's endogenous analgesics. Additionally, the rhythmic pressure of massage helps to improve circulation, enhance lymphatic drainage, and facilitate the removal of toxins from the body, further promoting relaxation and well-being.

Moreover, topical application is efficient for skincare, offering a natural and holistic approach to nourishing and rejuvenating the skin. Essential oils such as rosehip, frankincense, and geranium are renowned for their skin-healing and anti-aging features. These oils can lessen inflammation, encourage cellular regeneration, and hydrate and moisturize the skin when applied topically. Research has shown that essential oils contain compounds such as antioxidants, vitamins, and fatty acids, which help to protect against free radical damage, increase the formation of collagen and enhance the tone and texture of the skin. Additionally, essential oils have antimicrobial properties, effectively combating acne, blemishes, and other skin conditions. Individuals can naturally nourish and protect their skin by incorporating essential oils into skincare routines, promoting a healthy and radiant complexion.

Furthermore, topical essential oils offer targeted relief for many physical ailments and health concerns. Essential oils with antibacterial, analgesic, and anti-inflammatory qualities, such tea tree, eucalyptus, and peppermint, are perfect for minor wounds, scrapes, and insect bites. These oils, when applied topically, can aid in wound cleansing, pain and swelling reduction, and accelerated healing. Additionally, essential oils such as ginger, black pepper, and marjoram effectively relieve joint pain, muscle stiffness, and arthritis symptoms. Research has shown that topical application of these oils can help to increase circulation, reduce inflammation, and alleviate pain by blocking pain signals in the nervous system. By applying essential oils directly to affected areas, individuals can experience targeted relief for various physical ailments, promoting comfort and well-being.

Moreover, topical application of essential oils offers emotional support and promotes mental well-being. From ancient times, people have utilized essential oils with uplifting and stress-relieving effects, like bergamot, ylang-ylang, and clary sage. These oils, when used topically, can aid in emotional balance, anxiety reduction, and relaxation.Research has shown that essential oils contain compounds such as monoterpenes and sesquiterpenes, which help to regulate neurotransmitter activity in the brain, including the release of serotonin and dopamine—neurotransmitters associated with mood and emotions. Additionally, massaging essential oils into the skin helps advance relaxation, reduce stress, and enhance feelings of well-being by stimulating the release of oxytocin—the "love hormone" which is responsible for feelings of bonding and connection. By incorporating essential oils into massage and skincare routines, individuals can experience the therapeutic benefits of aromatherapy and promote overall health and vitality.

In conclusion, topical application of essential oils through massage and skincare offers many physical, emotional, and mental benefits. Topical application is a flexible and useful way to use the therapeutic qualities of essential oils, since it can be used to enhance general health, relieve muscle tension, and promote relaxation. By incorporating essential oils into daily self-care routines, individuals can experience the transformative power of aromatherapy and promote health, vitality, and balance in their lives. Whether through massage, skincare, or targeted relief for physical ailments, the topical application offers a natural and holistic approach to wellness, allowing individuals to connect with the healing power of nature and promote holistic well-being.

Diffusion: Creating Ambiance and Atmosphere

There are a lot of ways to diffuse essential oils in order to create atmosphere and ambience at home. However, there is one common way to use essential oils in aromatherapy which is through diffusion. It is releasing the aromatic molecules of the oils into the air to produce a relaxing and healing environment. This technique utilizes devices such as diffusers, nebulizers, and humidifiers to release essential oil vapors into the surrounding environment, allowing for easy inhalation and absorption of their therapeutic benefits. Diffusion offers many benefits for physical and emotional well- being, making it a versatile and practical approach to enhancing the ambiance and atmosphere of any space.

One of the primary benefits of diffusion is its ability to purify and freshen the air, creating a clean and refreshing environment. Natural antibacterial qualities of essential oils, such as those of tea tree, eucalyptus, and lemon, aid in the removal of airborne infections, the neutralization of odors, and the enhancement of a clean feeling. Diffusing essential oils is a useful way to promote respiratory health and avoid disease because research has shown that it can help lower levels of airborne germs and viruses. Diffusion also helps to purge the air of stale or disagreeable smells, replacing them with the invigorating scent of essential oils, which makes any space in the house feel cozy and welcoming.

Moreover, diffusion is highly effective for promoting relaxation and reducing stress, creating a soothing and tranquil ambiance that supports overall well-being. Essential oils with relaxing and anxiety-reducing qualities, such as lavender, chamomile, and bergamot, are perfect for diffusing in bedrooms, meditation areas, and relaxation places. When inhaled, these oils interact with olfactory receptors in the nasal cavity, triggering the release of neurotransmitters such as serotonin and dopamine, which are associated with feelings of relaxation and happiness. Additionally, diffusion helps to create a sense of serenity and peace by filling the air with the gentle aroma of essential oils, promoting relaxation and stress relief in individuals seeking to unwind and rejuvenate.

Furthermore, diffusion is a versatile and convenient method for having the therapeutic benefits of essential oils throughout the day. Whether at home, in the office, or while traveling, diffusers provide a continuous and consistent release of essential oil vapors, allowing for effortless inhalation and absorption of their healing properties. This makes diffusion an ideal choice for individuals seeking natural remedies for various health concerns, from promoting respiratory health and relaxation to improving mood and enhancing focus. Additionally, diffusers come in multiple styles and designs, allowing individuals to customize their aromatherapy experience to suit their preferences and lifestyle needs.

Additionally, diffusion is a safe and gentle method for administering essential oils, making it suitable for people of all ages and health conditions. Unlike topical application or ingestion, diffusion does not require direct contact with the skin or ingestion of the oils, making it a low-risk option for individuals with sensitive skin or gastrointestinal issues. Moreover, diffusion allows for a controlled and gradual release of essential oil vapors into the air, minimizing the risk of adverse reactions or overexposure. It makes diffusion an accessible and convenient option for individuals seeking to incorporate aromatherapy into their daily routines and promote health and well-being naturally.

In a nutshell, diffusion offers many benefits for creating ambiance and atmosphere while promoting physical, emotional, and mental well-being. From purifying the air and reducing stress to promoting relaxation and enhancing mood, diffusion provides a convenient and effective method for enjoying the therapeutic benefits of essential oils in any space. By incorporating diffusion into daily routines, individuals can experience the transformative power of aromatherapy and create a serene and inviting atmosphere that promotes health, happiness, and harmony. Whether at home, in the workplace, or while traveling, diffusion offers a natural and holistic approach to enhancing the ambiance and atmosphere of any environment, allowing individuals to connect with the healing power of nature and promote holistic well-being.

Bathing: Soaking in Aromatic Bliss

Essential oils have transformed bathing, a long-practiced custom in many cultures, into a therapeutic experience that offers numerous advantages to the body and mind. This ancient practice combines water's cleansing properties with essential oils' healing properties, creating a sensory-rich environment that promotes relaxation, rejuvenation, and overall well-being. Whether enjoyed as a luxurious indulgence or a daily self-care ritual, aromatic baths offer many benefits, making them a popular and effective method for harnessing the therapeutic power of essential oils.

There is one of the primary benefits of aromatic baths which is their ability to build up relaxation and reduce stress, creating a soothing and tranquil environment that encourages the release of tension and creates a sense of calm. Aromatic baths benefit greatly from the relaxing and anxiety-reducing qualities of essential oils like lavender, chamomile, and sandalwood, which have long been valued for their qualities. These oils release their aromatic molecules into the steam when they are added to warm bathwater, where they are then absorbed through the skin and inhaled, resulting in a series of physiological reactions. Research indicates that taking an essential oil-infused bath can effectively relieve stress and support emotional balance by lowering cortisol levels, heart rate, and encouraging feelings of relaxation and well-being.

Moreover, aromatic baths offer therapeutic benefits for the skin, helping to nourish, hydrate, and rejuvenate the complexion while promoting overall skin health. Essential oils such as rosehip, geranium, and frankincense are renowned for their skin-healing and anti-aging properties, making them ideal for skincare routines. When added to bathwater, these oils penetrate the epidermal layers, delivering vitamins, antioxidants, and fatty acids that help to moisturize, repair, and protect the skin. Research has shown that soaking in a bath infused with essential oils can help to improve skin texture and tone, reduce inflammation, and promote cellular regeneration, resulting in a healthier, more radiant complexion. Additionally, the bath's warm water helps open pores and increase blood circulation, further enhancing the absorption of essential oil nutrients and promoting overall skin health.

Furthermore, aromatic baths offer therapeutic benefits for respiratory health, helping to clear congestion, soothe respiratory symptoms, and promote easier breathing. Essential oils with decongestant, expectorant, and antibacterial qualities, such as eucalyptus, peppermint, and tea tree, have been utilized for respiratory treatment for a long time. These oils expand airways, lessen inflammation, and stop the growth of germs and viruses when they are added to bathwater. The aromatic molecules in the steam are then inhaled and absorbed through the sinuses, lungs, and nasal passages. Research indicates that taking an essential oil-infused bath can effectively alleviate symptoms of sinusitis, congestion, and coughing. This makes the bath a useful treatment for respiratory infections and respiratory health promotion.

Additionally, aromatic baths offer therapeutic benefits for promoting detoxification and supporting overall health and wellness. Essential oils such as juniper, grapefruit, and lemon include natural detoxifying properties that help cleanse the body of toxins, impurities, and metabolic waste, making them ideal for detox baths. These oils, when added to bathwater, aid in lymphatic drainage, circulation stimulation, and the body's natural detoxification processes—all of which aid in the removal of toxins and the enhancement of general health and vigor. Studies have indicated that taking an essential oil-infused bath can help to lower inflammation, promote circulation, and assist the body's natural detoxification processes. These advantages may result in improved digestion, more energy, and general wellbeing.

Taking everything into account, aromatic baths offer a luxurious and therapeutic experience that promotes relaxation, rejuvenation, and overall well-being. Whether enjoyed as a daily self-care ritual or an occasional indulgence, aromatic baths provide numerous benefits for both body and mind, making them a popular and effective method for harnessing the therapeutic power of essential oils. By incorporating aromatic baths into daily routines, individuals can experience the transformative effects of aromatherapy, promoting relaxation, skin health, respiratory wellness, and detoxification in the comfort of their homes. Whether seeking stress relief, skincare benefits, respiratory support, or detoxification, aromatic baths offer a natural and holistic approach to enhancing health and well-being, allowing individuals to immerse themselves in aromatic bliss and reap the benefits of this ancient and time-honored practice.

CHAPTER V

Aromatherapy for Everyday Wellness

Stress Relief and Relaxation

In the hectic and fast-paced world of today, stress is a common problem that affects millions of people globally. Prolonged stress can be harmful to one's physical and emotional well-being, resulting in a variety of symptoms like anxiety, sadness, sleeplessness, and even long-term conditions like diabetes and heart disease. Thus, developing efficient coping mechanisms and relaxation techniques is crucial for general health. Aromatherapy is one of such method that has become well-known for its capacity to lower tension and promote relaxation.

Utilizing plant-based essential oils, aromatherapy provides a holistic and all-natural method of relieving stress and promoting relaxation. Strong aromatic chemicals found in essential oils interact with the brain and olfactory system to cause a range of physiological and psychological reactions. These aromatic compounds have the ability to promote relaxation. It can regulate the neurological system, and modulate the body's stress response when applied topically or breathed.

Inhaling essential oils is one of the main ways aromatherapy encourages relaxation and stress alleviation. The therapeutic advantages of essential oils may be directly and effectively delivered to the brain by inhalation, where they can work their relaxing and mood-enhancing magic. Reputable for their ability to relieve stress, essential oils including lavender, chamomile, and bergamot can lower anxiety, boost relaxation, and enhance the quality of sleep. According to research, breathing in these oils can help lower cortisol levels, which are the body's main stress hormone, as well as heart rate, calmness, and peace.

Furthermore, aromatherapy encourages relaxation by influencing the limbic system, which is the part of the brain in charge of controlling emotions and stress reactions. Volatile substances found in essential oils have the capacity to cross the blood-brain barrier and influence brain neurotransmitter function, including the release of dopamine and serotonin. Modulation of these neurotransmitters can contribute to feelings of well-being and relaxation. These neurotransmitters are essential for controlling mood, emotions, and stress responses. The body's natural painkillers, endorphins, are also released when essential oils are inhaled, which helps to further induce relaxation and lower stress levels.

Additionally, aromatherapy encourages relaxation by influencing the autonomic nervous system, which controls involuntary body processes including digestion, blood pressure, and heart rate. Essential oils like lavender, rose, and sandalwood have shown that they can calm the autonomic nervous system by increasing parasympathetic activity (the "rest and digest" response) and reducing sympathetic activity (the "fight or flight" reaction). This change in autonomic balance mitigates the physiological impacts of stress, such as elevated heart rate and shallow breathing, and encourages relaxation. Studies have indicated that breathing in these oils can lower blood pressure, lower heart rate, and encourage general relaxation.

Additionally, aromatherapy helps people relax by influencing the endocrine system, which controls the release of chemicals that are essential for stress reactions. It has been demonstrated that adaptogenic essential oils, such as frankincense, vetiver, and ylang-

ylang, can regulate the discharge of stress hormones such as cortisol and adrenaline. These oils have the potential to boost general well-being, increase resilience to stress, and foster a sense of peace and relaxation by modulating the body's stress response. Furthermore, doing aromatherapy rituals like diffusing, topically applying, or taking aromatic baths can help foster a sense of routine and awareness that lowers stress and encourages relaxation.

In summary, aromatherapy promotes emotional well-being and restores physical and mental equilibrium while providing a safe, effective, and natural method of stress relief and relaxation. The intake or topical application of essential oils can provide people with the therapeutic advantages of aromatherapy, such as stress reduction, mood elevation, and increased relaxation. Through the integration of aromatherapy into regular self-care regimens, people can enhance their quality of life, develop stress resilience, and promote general well-being. Aromatherapy is a comprehensive method of managing stress that enables people to take charge of their health and well-being in a natural way. It can be used diffusely, topically, or in soothing baths.

Sleep Support and Insomnia Relief

In the current fast-paced and demanding world, stress has become prevalent, affecting millions all around the world. Prolonged stress can be harmful to one's physical and emotional well-being, resulting in a variety of symptoms like anxiety, sadness, sleeplessness, and even long-term conditions like diabetes and heart disease. Therefore, finding effective strategies to manage stress and promote relaxation is essential for overall well-being. One of these approaches that has gained widespread acceptance for its ability to reduce stress and induce relaxation is aromatherapy.

Aromatherapy, using essential oils derived from plants, suggest a natural and holistic way to stress relief and relaxation. Essential oils contain potent aromatic compounds that interact with the olfactory system and the brain, triggering a cascade of physiological and psychological responses. During inhalation or applying to the skin, these aromatic molecules can help modulate the body's stress response, promote relaxation, and restore balance to the nervous system.

One of the primary ways aromatherapy promotes stress relief and relaxation is by inhaling essential oils. Inhalation is a direct and efficient method for delivering the therapeutic benefits of essential oils to the brain, where they exert their calming and mood-enhancing effects. Reputable for their ability to relieve stress, essential oils such as lavender, chamomile, and bergamot can lower anxiety, encourage relaxation, and enhance the quality of sleep. Research has shown that inhaling these oils can help lower cortisol levels—the body's primary stress hormone—reduce heart rate, and promote calm and tranquility.

Moreover, aromatherapy promotes relaxation through its effects on the limbic system—the brain area responsible for regulating emotions and stress responses. Volatile substances found in essential oils have the capability to pass over the blood-brain barrier and influence brain neurotransmitter function, including the release of dopamine and serotonin. Modulation of these neurotransmitters can contribute to feelings of well-being and relaxation. These neurotransmitters are essential for controlling mood, emotions, and stress responses. Additionally, inhaling essential oils stimulates the release of endorphins—the body's natural painkillers—which further promote relaxation and reduce stress.

Additionally, aromatherapy encourages relaxation by influencing the autonomic nervous system, which controls involuntary body processes including digestion, blood pressure, and heart rate. The autonomic nervous system has been demonstrated to be calmed by essential oils including lavender, rose, and sandalwood, which serve to raise parasympathetic activity (the "rest and digest" response) and decrease sympathetic activity (the "fight or flight" reaction). This change in autonomic balance mitigates the physiological impacts of stress, such elevated heart rate and shallow breathing, and encourages relaxation. Studies have indicated that breathing in these oils can lower blood pressure, lower heart rate, and encourage general relaxation.

Additionally, aromatherapy helps people relax by influencing the endocrine system, which controls the release of chemicals that are essential for stress reactions. It has been demonstrated that adaptogenic essential oils, such frankincense, vetiver, and ylang-ylang, can regulate the clemency of stress hormones such as cortisol and adrenaline. By regulating the body's stress response, these oils can help promote a sense of calm and relaxation, improve resilience to stress, and enhance overall well-being. Additionally, engaging in aromatherapy rituals, such as diffusing essential oils, applying them topically, or enjoying aromatic baths, can help create a sense of ritual and mindfulness that promotes relaxation and reduces stress.

In conclusion, aromatherapy offers a natural and practical approach to stress relief and relaxation, promoting emotional well-being and restoring balance to the body and mind. When inhaling or appling topicaly essential oils, some people say that they can experience the therapeutic benefits of aromatherapy, including reduced stress, improved mood, and enhanced relaxation. By incorporating aromatherapy into daily self-care routines, individuals can cultivate resilience to stress, promote overall well-being, and improve quality of life. Whether through diffusing calming essential oils, applying them topically, or enjoying aromatic baths, aromatherapy offers a holistic approach to stress management that empowers individuals to take control of their health and well-being naturally.

Boosting Immunity and Fighting Infections

Boosting immunity and fighting infections are essential to maintaining overall health and well-being, especially in today's world, where threats from pathogens and diseases are ever-present. The immune system is the body's defense mechanism, protecting against harmful invaders like bacteria, viruses, and fungi. However, stress, poor nutrition, lack of sleep, and exposure to environmental toxins can impair immunity, increasing susceptibility to illnesses and illnesses. Therefore, finding effective strategies for enhancing immunity and supporting the body's natural defenses is crucial for preventing diseases and promoting optimal health.

One of the most effective ways to boost immunity is by adopting a healthy lifestyle which combine regular exercise, a balanced diet, adequate sleep, and stress management. Regular physical activity has been proved to have numerous benefits for immune function, including increasing the production of immune cells, improving circulation, and reducing inflammation. It was proven including activities such as walking, jogging, swimming, or yoga can help to better the immune system and improve tootal health and well-being . Furthermore, you can obtain essential nutrients like antioxidants, vitamins, and minerals which enchance your immune system and protect you from disease by eating a well-adjusted diet which includes fruits, vegetables, whole grains, and lean proteins. Foods high in immune-boosting nutrients, like citrus fruits, berries, garlic, ginger, and leafy greens, can assist to fortify the body's defenses against infections.

Furthermore, managing stress and promoting relaxation are essential for helping immune function and reducing the risk of infections. Constant stress has been shown to suppress immune function, making the body more susceptible to diseases and illnesses. Which is why, identifying healthy ways to cope with stress, such as practicing mindfulness meditation, deep breathing exercises, or devoting time to nature, can help reduce stress's adverse effects on the immune system and promote overall well-being. Additionally, ensuring adequate sleep is crucial for immune function, as sleep plays a key role in regulating immune responses and promoting healing and repair processes in the body. Some people can support immune function and reduce the risk of infections and illnesses by prioritizing sleep and implementing healthy sleep habits.

Moreover, incorporating immune-boosting herbs and supplements into one's diet can help to strengthen the body's natural defenses and enhance immunity. Certain herbs, such as echinacea, elderberry, and astragalus, have been used for centuries as natural remedies for boosting immunity and fighting infections. These herbs contain antiviral, antibacterial, and immune-stimulating compounds which help to support immune function and reduce the severity and duration of infections. Additionally, vitamins and minerals such as vitamin C, vitamin D, zinc, and probiotics play essential roles in immune function and can help to support the body's natural defenses against pathogens. Whether taken as dietary supplements or incorporated into the diet through food sources, these immune-boosting herbs and nutrients offer a natural and effective way to enhance immunity and protect against infections.

Furthermore, incorporating immune-boosting essential oils into one's daily routine can help to strengthen the body's natural defenses and promote overall health and well-being. Strong antibacterial qualities found in essential oils including thyme, oregano, eucalyptus, and tea tree can aid in the prevention of infections and boost immune system performance. Whether these immune-boosting oils are used to homemade cleaning products, diffused, or applied topically, they provide a safe and efficient means of warding off infections and advancing well-being. In addition, applying essential oils like frankincense, lavender, and chamomile can boost general well-being by lowering stress, encouraging relaxation, and strengthening the immune system while lowering the risk of infections and illnesses.

In a nutshell, maintaining general health and well-being requires enhancing immunity and preventing infections, particularly in the modern world where germs and diseases provide a constant threat. People can strengthen their immune systems and reduce their risk of infections and disease by adopting healthy behaviors such as stress management, regular exercise, adequate sleep, and a well-balanced diet. Additionally, incorporating immune-boosting herbs, supplements, and essential oils into one's daily routine which can further support immune function and promote optimal health and wellness. By prioritizing immune health and implementing healthy habits, individuals can enhance their body's natural defenses and enjoy a greater sense of vitality and well-being.

Managing Pain and Discomfort

Managing pain and discomfort is a universal challenge, whether due to acute injuries, chronic conditions, or everyday aches and pains. Conventional therapies, such as medicine and physical therapy, may have drawbacks and adverse consequences in addition to their potential effectiveness. As a result, many people are turning to natural and holistic approaches to pain management, including the use of aromatherapy. Aromatherapy, the therapeutic use of essential oils came from plants, offers a gentle and versatile approach to managing pain and discomfort, relieving many conditions while promoting overall well-being.

One of the primary ways aromatherapy manages pain and discomfort is through its analgesic and anti-inflammatory properties. Essential oils contain volatile aromatic compounds that have been shown to have pain-relieving and anti-inflammatory effects, making them effective remedies for alleviating various types of pain, including muscle soreness, joint pain, and headaches. Essential oils with analgesic qualities, such lavender, eucalyptus, and peppermint, have long been used topically or breathed to lessen the length and intensity of pain. Research has shown that these oils can help inhibit pain signals, reduce inflammation, and promote relaxation, making them practical options for managing acute and chronic pain.

Moreover, aromatherapy manages pain and discomfort through its effects on the central nervous system, which is crucial in processing pain signals and regulating pain perception. There are essential oils such as frankincense, ginger, and helichrysum have been shown to have modulating effects on neurotransmitter activity in the brain, helping to relieve pain sensitivity and increase pain tolerance. By inhaling or applying these oils topically, individuals can help alleviate pain symptoms and promote a sense of comfort and well-being. To further improve pain management, aromatherapy practices like diffusing essential oils throughout the house or rubbing them into afflicted regions can help create a relaxing and pleasant atmosphere that encourages relaxation and lowers stress.

Furthermore, aromatherapy manages pain and discomfort through its impact on the autonomic nervous system, which is responsible for regulating involuntary bodily functions that includes heart rate, blood pressure, and digestion. Essential oils including chamomile, clary sage, and rosemary have been shown to have calming and soothing effects on the autonomic nervous system, helping to cut down sympathetic activity (the "fight or flight" response) and increase parasympathetic activity (the "rest and digest" response). This shift in autonomic balance promotes relaxation and reduces muscle tension, which can help to alleviate pain symptoms and improve overall comfort. Additionally, engaging in aromatherapy rituals, such as taking aromatic baths or applying essential oils to pulse points, can help create a sense of ritual and mindfulness that promotes relaxation and enhances pain relief.

Moreover, aromatherapy manages pain and discomfort through its effects on emotional well-being, which plays a crucial role in pain perception and coping mechanisms. Essential oils such as bergamot, geranium, and ylang-ylang have been shown to have mood-enhancing and stress-reducing effects, helping to promote a positive outlook and improve coping skills. By using these oils or applying them topically, individuals can help alleviate emotional distress and promote feelings of calm and relaxation, reducing pain intensity and improving overall comfort. Additionally, engaging in aromatherapy rituals, such as diffusing essential oils or practicing aromatherapy massage, can help build a nurturing and supportive environment that promotes emotional well-being and enhances pain relief.

In summary, aromatherapy relieves a variety of ailments and enhances general wellbeing. It is a natural, safe, and efficient way to deal with pain and suffering. Individuals may profit from the medicinal properties of aromatherapy, such as pain alleviation, inflammation reduction, and mental support, by inhaling or using essential oils topically. By incorporating aromatherapy into daily self-care routines, individuals can cultivate resilience to pain, improve coping skills, and enhance overall quality of life. Whether through diffusing pain-relieving essential oils, applying them topically to affected areas, or enjoying aromatic baths, aromatherapy offers a holistic approach to pain management that empowers individuals to take control of their health and well-being naturally.

CHAPTER VI

Integrating Aromatherapy into Daily Life

How to Create Aromatic Spaces in Your Home

Creating aromatic spaces in your home is a delightful and effective way to enhance the ambiance, promote relaxation, and enhance general health. The therapeutic application of plant-derived essential oils, or aromatherapy, offers a natural and versatile approach to infusing your living environment with delightful scents while reaping the numerous benefits of aromatherapy. Incorporating essential oils into various aspects of your home decor and daily routines allows you to create inviting and soothing spaces that promote relaxation, reduce stress, and uplift the mood.

Essential oil diffusers are one of the simplest ways to create aromatic spaces in your home. Essential oils are released into the air by diffusers, enabling you to enjoy their fragrant qualities throughout your house. Several types of diffusers are available, including ultrasonic diffusers, nebulizing diffusers, and passive diffusers, each offering unique benefits and features. Nebulizing diffusers employ compressed air to break down essential oils into tiny particles for inhalation, while ultrasonic diffusers use water to distribute essential oils into the air as a fine mist. Passive diffusers, such as reed and aromatherapy jewelry, release essential oils into the air through evaporation, providing a subtle and continuous fragrance.

In addition to diffusers, you can create aromatic spaces in your home using scented candles, potpourri, and room sprays. Essential oil-infused scented candles provide a comforting aroma that can turn any space into a comfortable haven. Choose candles with cotton wicks and soy wax instead of synthetic ones to reduce your exposure to dangerous chemicals. Potpourri, made from dried flowers, herbs, and spices infused with essential oils, adds a decorative touch to any room while releasing a subtle and long-lasting fragrance. Room sprays, made from a blend of water, alcohol, and essential oils, provide a quick and convenient way to refresh and invigorate any space.

Moreover, you can create aromatic spaces in your home by using aromatic baths and showers. You may create a revitalizing and soothing spa-like atmosphere with a few drops of essential oil added to the water in your bath or shower. Because they are so soothing and revitalizing, essential oils like eucalyptus, lavender, and chamomile are especially good for baths and showers. To experience the healing powers of aromatherapy, a few drops of your favorite essential oil should be added to a warm bath or a damp washcloth, then take a deep breath. Furthermore, you can create aromatic spaces in your home using natural cleaning products infused with essential oils.

Numerous cleaning products for business use include strong chemicals and synthetic fragrances that can cause indoor air pollution and aggravate the respiratory system. Essential oils, vinegar, and baking soda are examples of natural substances that can be mixed to create cleaning solutions that efficiently clean and freshen your house without putting you in danger of harmful chemicals. Essential oils with antibacterial and antiviral qualities, like lemon, tea tree, and peppermint, are perfect for use in cleaning products.

Additionally, you can create aromatic spaces in your home using aromatherapy spritzers and linen sprays. These homemade sprays can be made using distilled water and a few drops of your favorite essential oils, creating a refreshing and uplifting fragrance that can be sprayed on bedding, curtains, upholstery, and clothing. Essential oils such as lavender rose and bergamot are particularly well-suited for spritzers and linen sprays due to their calming properties. Mix the essential oils with distilled water in a spray bottle and shake well before each use to enjoy the aromatic benefits of aromatherapy.

In conclusion, creating aromatic spaces in your home is a simple and effective way to enhance the ambiance, promote relaxation, and improve overall well-being. Incorporating essential oils into various aspects of your home decor and daily routines allows you to create inviting and soothing spaces that uplift the mood and reduce stress. Whether using diffusers, scented candles, aromatic baths, natural cleaning products, or homemade spritzers, aromatherapy offers a versatile and enjoyable approach to infusing your living environment with delightful scents and therapeutic benefits. Experiment with different essential oils and diffusion methods to discover the perfect aromatic blend for your home, and enjoy the transformative effects of aromatherapy on your health and happiness.

Aromatherapy in the Workplace: Enhancing Productivity and Well-being

Aromatherapy in the workplace has emerged as a popular and effective strategy for enhancing productivity, reducing stress, and promoting overall employee well- being. In today's fast-paced and demanding work environments, employees often face high stress, fatigue, and burnout, which can have a detrimental effect on their output, happiness at work, and morale. Aromatherapy provides a safe, natural method to address these challenges, providing employees with a sensory experience that can help to create a more positive and supportive work environment.

One of the primary ways aromatherapy enhances productivity and well-being in the workplace is through its ability to reduce tension and unease. Essential oils with calming and relaxing qualities, such bergamot, chamomile, and lavender, are well known for their ability to support a sense of calm and tranquility. By diffusing these oils in the workplace, employers can establish a serene and stress-free atmosphere that helps employees unwind and recharge during busy workdays. Research has shown that inhaling these oils can help to reduce cortisol levels—the body's primary stress hormone—lower blood pressure and promote feelings of relaxation and wellbeing, which enhances output and contentment at work.

Moreover, aromatherapy enhances productivity and well-being in the workplace by improving cognitive function and mental clarity. Essential oils with well-known properties include peppermint, rosemary, and lemon.stimulating and invigorating properties, helping to boost alertness, concentration, and memory retention. By diffusing these oils in the workplace, employers can create an exciting and energizing environment that allows employees to stay focused and productive throughout the day. Research has shown that inhaling these oils can help to improve cognitive performance, enhance mental clarity, and reduce mental fatigue, leading to improved productivity and job performance.

Furthermore, aromatherapy enhances productivity and well-being in the workplace by promoting physical health and reducing sick days. Essential oils including eucalyptus, tea tree, and cinnamon have antibacterial, antiviral, and immune-boosting properties that help to cut down the spread of germs and pathogens in the workplace. By diffusing these oils in the workplace, employers can produce a clean and hygienic environment headwear hinders the transmission of disease and reduce the risk of absenteeism. Research has shown that inhaling these oils can aid in boosting immunity, lower the chance of respiratory infections, as well as enhance general health and wellbeing, which reduces the need for sick days and increases output.

Moreover, aromatherapy enhances productivity and well-being in the workplace by improving mood and morale. Essential oils such as citrus, lavender, and geranium are known for their mood-enhancing and uplifting properties, helping promote a positive and supportive work environment. By diffusing these oils in the workplace, employers may produce a happy and inviting environment that makes employees feel happier and more motivated. Research has shown that inhaling these oils can help to increase serotonin and dopamine levels—the "feel-good" neurotransmitters—in the brain, leading to improved mood and morale, higher job satisfaction, and reduced turnover rates.

Additionally, aromatherapy enhances productivity and well-being in the workplace by promoting relaxation and stress management techniques. Many companies offer aromatherapy workshops or relaxation sessions as part of their employee wellness programs, allowing employees to learn about the benefits of aromatherapy and how to incorporate it into their daily routines. By teaching employees how to use essential oils safely and effectively, employers can empower them to take control of their health and well-being and reduce stress levels in and out of the workplace. Research has shown that participating in aromatherapy workshops can help reduce stress, improve sleep quality, and enhance overall well-being, leading to higher productivity and job satisfaction.

Finally, aromatherapy provides a safe and efficient means of enhancing productivity and well-being in the workplace, providing employees with a sensory encounter that enhances general health, eases tension, and encourages relaxation happiness. By diffusing essential oils in the workplace, employers may foster a climate that is encouraging and helpful, employees feel happier, more focused, and more motivated. Whether through calming oils to reduce stress, stimulating oils to boost cognitive function, or immune-boosting oils to promote physical health, aromatherapy offers a versatile and enjoyable approach to enhancing productivity and wellbeing at work. Companies can cultivate a more contented, robust, and efficient workforce by incorporating aromatherapy into their employee wellness programs.

Traveling with Essential Oils: Tips for Healthier Journeys

While traveling can be a fascinating and rewarding experience, it can also affect our physical and mental well-being. Long flights, cramped seats, unfamiliar environments, and jet lag can leave us energized, relaxed, and balanced. Thankfully, essential oils provide a safe, all-natural means of promoting our health and wellbeing when we're on the road. With their potent therapeutic properties, essential oils can help alleviate travel-related discomforts, boost immunity, and promote relaxation, making our journeys more enjoyable and rejuvenating. This section will explore the benefits of traveling with essential oils and provide tips for using them effectively to enhance your travel experience.

One of the primary benefits of traveling with essential oils is their ability to alleviate common travel-related discomforts such as nausea, motion sickness, and digestive issues. Essential oils such as ginger, peppermint, and spearmint are well-known for their anti-nausea and digestive properties. They are ideal remedies for alleviating nausea and stomach upset during flights or long car rides. Simply inhaling these oils or applying them to acupressure points such as the wrists or temples can help soothe the stomach and alleviate discomfort, allowing you to enjoy your journey without feeling queasy or nauseous.

Moreover, essential oils can help support our immune system and protect us from germs and pathogens while traveling. Strong antibacterial and antiviral qualities found in essential oils such as lavender, eucalyptus, and tea tree can help destroy bacteria and germs while enhancing our bodies' natural defenses against disease. You can lessen your chance of getting a cold or flu while traveling by diffusing essential oils in your hotel room or cabin to help filter the air and create a neat and hygienic environment. Applying these oils topically to pulse points or inhaling them directly can help support respiratory health and strengthen the immune system, ensuring you stay healthy and well throughout your journey.

Furthermore, essential oils can help promote relaxation and reduce stress and anxiety during travel. Essential oils that are known for their calming and soothing qualities, such as lavender, chamomile, and bergamot, can assist to promote peace and tranquility by relaxing the body and mind. Diffusing these oils in your hotel room or cabin can create a peaceful and restful environment that helps you unwind and relax after a long day of traveling. Additionally, applying these oils to pulse points or inhaling them directly can help reduce stress and anxiety and promote a sense of calm and well-being, allowing you to enjoy your journey with greater ease and relaxation.

Essential oils not only improve physical and mental health, but they can also make travel more enjoyable by evoking a multisensory experience that awakens all of our senses. Essential oils such as citrus oils, pine, and cedarwood can evoke memories of nature and the outdoors, helping to create a sense of adventure and exploration. Diffusing these oils in your hotel room or cabin can transport you to a peaceful forest or sunny citrus grove, providing a welcome escape from the hustle and bustle of travel. Applying these oils to pulse points or inhaling them directly can help invigorate the senses and uplift the mood, making your journey more enjoyable and memorable.

Moreover, essential oils can help alleviate jet lag and promote restful sleep during travel. Essential oils with calming qualities, such lavender, chamomile, and sandalwood, aid in body and mind relaxation and encourage sound sleep. After a tiring day of travel, diffuse these oils in your hotel room or cabin to create a calming and comfortable atmosphere that will help you wind down and get ready for bed. You can obtain the sleep you require to feel renewed and revitalized for your upcoming travels by applying these oils on your pulse points or immediately breathing them.

Furthermore, essential oils can help alleviate travel-related headaches, muscle aches, and tension. Essential oils with analgesic and anti-inflammatory qualities, such peppermint, eucalyptus, and rosemary, they can ease headache reduce soreness and reduce tense muscles from exertion or stress when traveling. Applying these oils topically to the temples, forehead, or sore muscles can provide immediate relief from pain and tension, allowing you to continue your journey with greater comfort and ease. Additionally, directly inhaling these oils can help reduce stress and tension and promote relaxation, enhancing their pain-relieving effects.

In conclusion, using essential oils when traveling is a safe, natural approach to maintain your health and wellbeing while you're on the go. Essential oils can provide valuable support and relief if you're looking to alleviate travel-related discomforts, boost immunity, promote relaxation, or enhance the overall travel experience. Traveling with essential oils can make your trip healthier, happier, and more pleasurable if you incorporate them into your routine and use them wisely. So next time you hit the road or take to the skies, remember to pack your essential oils and let their therapeutic properties help you travel with greater ease and comfort.

Aromatherapy for Special Occasions and Celebrations

Aromatherapy for special occasions and celebrations offers a unique and delightful way to enhance the ambiance, create memorable experiences, and promote emotional well-being among guests. Aromatherapy can be used to bring a touch of luxury, elegance, and customization to many areas of event planning and decor, from birthdays and weddings to holidays and anniversaries. By strategically selecting and diffusing essential oils that evoke specific emotions and memories, hosts can create an immersive sensory experience that delights the senses and leaves a lasting impression on guests.

One of the primary ways aromatherapy enhances special occasions, and celebrations are by creating signature scents that evoke the theme or mood of the event. Due to their seductive and enticing scents, essential oils like rose, jasmine, and ylang-ylang are popular options for romantic occasions like weddings. Hosts can create a romantic and enchanting atmosphere that sets the stage for love and romance by diffusing these oils throughout the venue or incorporating them into floral arrangements and centerpieces. Similarly, essential oils such as pine, cinnamon, and cedarwood are perfect for holiday gatherings and winter celebrations, as they evoke the cozy and festive spirit of the season.

Moreover, aromatherapy enhances special occasions and celebrations by promoting relaxation and reducing stress among guests. Essential oils with calming and soothing qualities, like bergamot, lavender, and chamomile, are well known for their ability to reduce stress, encourage relaxation, and foster a sense of peace. By diffusing these oils throughout the venue or incorporating them into massage oils and spa treatments, hosts can create a serene and peaceful atmosphere that helps guests unwind and de-stress. Additionally, providing guests with scented sachets or aromatherapy gifts to take home can extend the benefits of aromatherapy beyond the event and serve as a thoughtful reminder of the special occasion.

Furthermore, aromatherapy enhances special occasions and celebrations by evoking memories and creating emotional connections among guests. Essential oils can evoke powerful emotions and memories through unique fragrances, triggering associations with past experiences and personal connections. By selecting critical oils that hold special significance to the host or guests, such as their favorite scents or scents associated with meaningful memories, hosts can create a deeply personal and meaningful experience that resonates with everyone in attendance. Whether it's the scent of fresh flowers that reminds guests of a cherished garden or the smell of warm spices that evoke memories of holiday baking with loved ones, aromatherapy can help create a sense of nostalgia and connection that enhances the event's overall experience.

Additionally, aromatherapy enhances special occasions and celebrations by promoting physical health and well-being among guests. Strong antibacterial and immune-boosting qualities of essential oils, such those of tea tree, eucalyptus, and lemon, can support overall health and wellbeing by halting the transmission of bacteria and germs. By diffusing these oils throughout the venue or incorporating them into hand sanitizers and cleaning products, hosts can create a clean and hygienic environment that helps protect guests from illness and promotes a sense of safety and well-being. Additionally, offering guests aromatherapy treatments such as hand massages or inhalers can immediately relieve stress and tension and promote overall relaxation and well-being.

Moreover, aromatherapy enhances special occasions and celebrations by engaging the senses and creating a multi-sensory guest experience. In addition to diffusing essential oils, hosts can incorporate aromatherapy into various aspects of event planning and decor, such as scented candles, floral arrangements, and potpourri. By appealing to all five senses—sight, smell, taste, touch, and sound—hosts can create a fully immersive experience that captivates guests and leaves a lasting impression. Whether the scent of fresh flowers, the taste of aromatic cocktails, or the feel of luxurious essential oil-infused hand lotion, aromatherapy can help create a sensory journey that delights and enchants guests from start to finish.

Sum up the main points, aromatherapy offers a unique and versatile way to enhance special occasions and celebrations, creating memorable experiences that delight the senses and promote emotional well-being among guests. By incorporating essential oils into various aspects of event planning and decor, hosts can create a personalized and immersive experience that resonates with guests on a deep and meaningful level. Whether it's evoking the romance of a wedding, the festive spirit of the holidays, or the nostalgia of cherished memories, aromatherapy can elevate any special occasion and create lasting memories that guests will treasure for years.

CHAPTER VII

Aromatherapy for Emotional Healing

Addressing Anxiety and Depression

Addressing anxiety and depression is a critical aspect of mental health care, as these conditions affect millions of people worldwide and can have profound effects on individuals' quality of life. In addition to conventional therapies like counseling and medication, which are essential for controlling anxiety and depression, many people look for complementary and alternative methods to promote their mental health. Aromatherapy is one of the methods that has improved popularity due to its ability to promote emotional balance and well-being, alleviate anxiety and depressive symptoms, and employ essential oils obtained from plants therapeutically.

One of the primary ways in which aromatherapy can help address anxiety and depression is through its calming and stress-relieving properties. Fragrance oils like bergamot, lavender, and chamomile are well-known for their ability to soothe the nervous system and promote relaxation, making them effective remedies for reducing symptoms of anxiety and stress. Research has shown that inhaling these oils or applying them topically can help lower levels of cortisol—the body's primary stress hormone—and promote feelings of calm and tranquility. Additionally, these oils can help improve sleep quality and reduce insomnia, which are common symptoms of both anxiety and depression.

Moreover, aromatherapy can help address anxiety and depression by promoting a positive mood and emotional well-being. Essential oils such as citrus oils, rose, and geranium are known for their mood-enhancing properties, helping to uplift the spirits and promote feelings of happiness and contentment. Research has shown that inhaling these oils can help increase levels of serotonin and dopamine—the "feel-good" neurotransmitters—in the brain, leading to improved mood and reduced symptoms of depression. Additionally, these oils can help reduce feelings of agitation and irritability, which are common symptoms of anxiety and depression.

Furthermore, aromatherapy can help address anxiety and depression by promoting emotional release and healing. Essential oils such as frankincense, sandalwood, and vetiver are known for their grounding and centering properties, helping to calm the mind and promote emotional stability. Research has shown that inhaling these oils or applying them topically can help individuals process and release pent-up emotions, reducing feelings of anxiety and depression. Additionally, these oils can help individuals feel more connected to themselves and their feelings, facilitating a more profound sense of self-awareness and inner peace.

Additionally, aromatherapy can help address anxiety and depression by promoting self-care and stress management techniques. Many individuals find that incorporating aromatherapy into their daily self-care routines, such as through aromatherapy baths, massages, or diffusing essential oils throughout the home, can aid in lowering anxiety and depressive symptoms while enhancing general wellbeing. Studies have indicated that consistent self-care routines can improve mental health outcomes. Additionally, aromatherapy can serve as a mindfulness practice, assisting individuals to stay present and focused on the present moment, which can be beneficial for reducing anxiety and depression symptoms.

Moreover, aromatherapy can help address anxiety and depression by providing a sense of empowerment and control over one's mental health. Many individuals find that incorporating aromatherapy into their self-care routines gives them a sense of agency and autonomy over their well-being, allowing them to manage their symptoms and promote emotional balance actively. Furthermore, aromatherapy can be an affordable and easily accessible kind of mental health care, which makes it a desirable choice for people who might not have access to conventional treatments or who would rather take a more natural approach to wellbeing.

Summing up everything, aromatherapy offers a promising approach to addressing anxiety and depression, providing individuals with natural and practical tools to support their mental well-being. Using the medicinal qualities of essential oils, people can lessen their depressive and anxious symptoms. promote emotional balance and well-being, and enhance their overall quality of life. Aromatherapy can be a useful adjunct to current therapies, providing people with extra support and tools for managing their mental health, even if it shouldn't take the place of conventional treatments for anxiety and depression. As research in this area continues to grow, aromatherapy has the potential to play an increasingly important role in mental health care, helping individuals live happier, healthier, and more fulfilling lives.

Healing Trauma and Emotional Wounds

Healing trauma and emotional wounds is a complex and deeply personal journey that requires time, patience, and support. Numerous events, such as abuse, neglect, mishaps, natural disasters, and interpersonal conflicts, can lead to traumatic experiences. A person's physical, mental, and emotional well-being may be significantly and permanently impacted. While therapy and other forms of conventional treatment play a crucial role in healing trauma, many individuals also seek complementary and alternative approaches to support their recovery. One such method that has gained popularity is aromatherapy, which is the therapeutic application of essential oils obtained from plants. It has the ability to balance emotions, calm the nervous system, and aid in deep-level healing.

One of the primary ways aromatherapy can support healing trauma and emotional wounds is through its calming and grounding properties. Essential oils that are known to calm the nervous system and encourage relaxation, including lavender, chamomile, and frankincense, are useful treatments for lessening the feelings of anxiety, panic, and hypervigilance that are frequently connected to trauma. Research has shown that inhaling these oils or applying them topically can help lower levels of cortisol—the body's primary stress hormone—and promote feelings of calm and safety, creating a supportive environment for processing and integrating traumatic experiences.

Moreover, aromatherapy can support healing trauma and emotional wounds by facilitating emotional release and expression. Essential oils such as bergamot, rose, and geranium are known for their uplifting and heart-opening properties, helping to promote emotional healing and release pent-up emotions stored in the body. Research has shown that inhaling or using these oils in massage therapy can help individuals access and process deeply buried emotions, facilitating cathartic release and promoting a sense of emotional liberation. Additionally, these oils can help individuals feel more connected to themselves and their innermost feelings, fostering a deeper comprehension of acceptance and self-awareness.

Furthermore, aromatherapy can support healing trauma and emotional wounds by promoting self-care and self-nurturing practices. Many people claim that they have experienced trauma and struggle with feelings of worthlessness, shame, and self-doubt, making self-care activities challenging but essential for recovery. Incorporating aromatherapy into daily self-care routines, such as baths, massages, or diffusing essential oils throughout the home, can help individuals reconnect with their bodies, thoughts, and souls and foster a stronger feeling of self-love and compassion. Research has shown that engaging in regular self-care practices can help individuals rebuild a sense of trust and safety within themselves and create a supportive foundation for healing trauma and emotional wounds.

Additionally, aromatherapy can support healing trauma and emotional wounds by promoting a sense of empowerment and control over one's healing journey. Many individuals find that incorporating aromatherapy into their self-care routines gives them a sense of agency and autonomy over their healing process, allowing them to take an active role in their recovery and reclaim power over their lives. Additionally, aromatherapy can serve as a tangible and accessible tool for managing symptoms of trauma, providing people with a safe and natural way to soothe their nervous system, regulate their emotions, and find comfort and solace during difficult times.

Moreover, aromatherapy can support healing trauma and emotional wounds by fostering a sense of connection and community. Many individuals who have experienced trauma feel isolated and alone in their struggles, making it difficult to reach out for support or connect with others who understand their experiences. Participating in aromatherapy workshops, support groups, or online communities that can provide individuals with a safe and supportive space to share their stories, learn from others, and find solidarity and validation in their healing journey.

Additionally, engaging in aromatherapy practices with loved ones or trusted friends can strengthen bonds and foster a sense of belonging and acceptance, providing much-needed support and encouragement.

On a final note, aromatherapy offers a valuable and holistic approach to healing trauma and emotional wounds, providing individuals with natural and practical tools to support their recovery and promote emotional well-being. Through the application of essential oils' therapeutic qualities, people can promote self-nurturing and self-care behaviors that deeply promote healing, relax their nerve systems, and enable emotional release. While aromatherapy should not replace conventional treatments for trauma, it can serve as a valuable complement to therapy and other forms of support, offering individuals additional resources and tools for managing symptoms and reclaiming their lives. As research in this area continues to grow, aromatherapy has the potential to play an increasingly important role in trauma recovery, helping individuals heal from the inside out and reclaim a sense of peace, wholeness, and resilience.

Cultivating Emotional Resilience with Aromatherapy

Cultivating emotional resilience is crucial for navigating life's challenges and setbacks with grace and strength. The ability to adjust to pressures, overcome hardship, and preserve equilibrium and well-being in the face of adversity is referred to as emotional resilience. Even though some people may be more emotionally resilient by nature than others, emotional resilience is a talent that can be strengthened and developed over time with deliberate practice. Aromatherapy, the therapeutic application of essential oils derived from plants, offers a unique and successful method for building emotional resilience by reducing stress and promoting relaxation, inner harmony, and quiet.

We have one of the primary ways aromatherapy which can support the cultivation of emotional resilience. It is done by reducing stress and promoting relaxation. Essential oils with calming and soothing qualities, like bergamot, chamomile, and lavender, are proven to ease tension and anxiety by calming the body and mind. Research has shown that inhaling or using these oils in massage therapy can help lower cortisol levels—the body's primary stress hormone—and promote deep relaxation, allowing individuals to recharge and rejuvenate their energy reserves. Additionally, these oils can help improve sleep quality and reduce insomnia, which are common symptoms of chronic stress and burnout.

Moreover, aromatherapy can support emotional resilience by promoting emotional release and healing. Essential oils with grounding and centering qualities, including frankincense, rose, and sandalwood, are believed to support emotional stability and assist the discharge of emotions that have been trapped in the body. Research has shown that inhaling or using these oils in aromatherapy baths or massages can help individuals access and process deeply buried emotions, allowing them to release emotional baggage and find closure and healing from past traumas or hardships. Additionally, these oils can help individuals feel more connected to themselves and their emotions, fostering a greater sense of self-awareness and acceptance.

Furthermore, aromatherapy can support the cultivation of emotional resilience by promoting self-care and self-nurturing practices. Burnout and exhaustion can result from many people who struggle with emotional resilience, prioritizing the needs of others over their own. Incorporating aromatherapy into daily self-care routines, such as baths, massages, or diffusing essential oils throughout the home, can help individuals reconnect with their bodies, brains, and spirits and develop a stronger feeling of compassion and self-love. Studies have indicated that consistent self-care routines can help individuals build emotional resilience and better cope with stress and adversity, improving mental and emotional well-being.

Additionally, aromatherapy can support emotional resilience by fostering a sense of empowerment and control over one's emotional well-being. Many individuals who struggle with emotional resilience may feel helpless or overwhelmed by their emotions, leading to feelings of anxiety and depression. Incorporating aromatherapy into their self-care routines gives them a tangible and accessible tool for managing their feelings and promoting emotional balance and well-being. By choosing and using essential oils that resonate with their needs and preferences, individuals can take an active role in their emotional healing journey, reclaiming power and agency over their lives.

Moreover, aromatherapy can support emotional resilience by fostering a sense of connection and community. Many individuals who struggle with emotional resilience may feel isolated and alone in their struggles, making it difficult to reach out for support or connect with others who understand their experiences. A safe and encouraging environment may be found for people to share their stories, learn from others, and receive support and validation in their journey toward emotional resilience by taking part in aromatherapy workshops, support groups, or online communities. Additionally, engaging in aromatherapy practices with loved ones or trusted friends can strengthen bonds and foster a sense of belonging and acceptance, providing much-needed support and encouragement.

In conclusion, aromatherapy offers a valuable and holistic approach to cultivating emotional resilience. It provides individuals with natural and practical tools to support their emotional well-being and navigate life's challenges with greater ease and grace. Through the utilization of essential oils' therapeutic qualities, people can provide a conducive atmosphere for developing emotional resilience by calming their nervous system, encouraging relaxation, and facilitating emotional release and healing.While aromatherapy should not replace professional therapy or other forms of support for emotional resilience, It can be a beneficial addition to current therapies, offering individuals additional resources and tools for managing their emotions and reclaiming their lives. As research in this area continues to grow, aromatherapy has the potential to play an increasingly important role in promoting emotional resilience and well-being, assisting people in leading more contented, healthy, and happy lives.

CHAPTER VIII

Aromatherapy for Specific Populations

Aromatherapy for Children and Babies

Aromatherapy for children and babies offers a gentle and natural approach to supporting their health and well-being from infancy through childhood. Essential oils are made from a variety of flowers and plants, contain potent therapeutic properties that can be harnessed to address common childhood ailments, promote relaxation, and enhance emotional and cognitive development. While aromatherapy can benefit children and babies, it is essential to approach its use cautiously and adopt safety guidelines to arrange their safety and well-being.

One of the primary ways aromatherapy can benefit children and babies is by supporting their respiratory health. Essential oils like eucalyptus, tea tree, and lavender have decongestant, antiviral, and antibacterial properties that help reduce the symptoms of colds, coughs, and respiratory infections. These oils can ease respiratory irritation and congestion by helping to unclog nasal passages, lessen inflammation, and make breathing easier. They can also be used topically in a diluted form and diffused into the air. However, it is crucial to use caution when diffusing essential oils around infants and young children, as their respiratory systems are still developing and may be more sensitive to strong fragrances.

Moreover, aromatherapy can benefit children and babies by promoting relaxation and better sleep quality. Essential oils that are considered to be calming and soothing, including frankincense, lavender, and chamomile, can help children of all ages feel less stressed, anxious, and restless. Use a few drops of these oils in a warm bath or diffuse them in the bedroom before bed to create a relaxing and peaceful environment that promotes restful sleep. Additionally, gentle massage with diluted essential oils can help relax tense muscles, promote circulation, and calm the nervous system, further enhancing relaxation and promoting a sense of well- being.

Furthermore, aromatherapy can benefit children and babies by supporting their emotional and cognitive development. Essential oils such as citrus, rosemary, and peppermint are known for their refreshing and uplifting properties, helping improve children's focus, concentration, and mental clarity. Diffusing these oils during study or playtime can help stimulate cognitive function, enhance memory retention, and promote a positive mood, making learning more enjoyable and engaging for children. Additionally, aromatherapy can help children and babies develop a positive association with self-care rituals, such as massage or bath time, fostering a sense of comfort and security that supports their emotional development.

Additionally, aromatherapy can benefit children and babies by supporting their immune systems and promoting overall health and well-being. Strong antibacterial and immune-stimulating qualities of essential oils, such as those found in tea tree, lemon, and thyme, can help guard against frequent childhood infections and diseases. Spreading these oils in the home or using homemade cleaning products can help purify the air, eliminate toxic microorganisms, and foster a more wholesome atmosphere that will enable infants and kids to flourish. Additionally, incorporating aromatherapy into daily self-care routines can help strengthen the bond between caregivers and children, fostering a sense of trust and security that supports their emotional and physical development.

However, it is essential to be cautious when using aromatherapy with children and babies, as their delicate systems may be more susceptible to adverse reactions. Therefore, before using essential oils topically, they must be adequately diluted because undiluted oils can irritate the skin or trigger allergic reactions. Additionally, using a lower concentration of essential oils when diffusing them in the air is recommended, especially in enclosed spaces where children and babies spend a lot of time. Since some essential oils can irritate the respiratory system, it is best to avoid using them on young children, especially peppermint and eucalyptus.

Taking everything into account aromatherapy is a safe, all-natural way to improve infants' and children's health and wellbeing, as well as to relieve common illnesses, encourage relaxation, and advance cognitive and emotional growth. When used safely and appropriately, essential oils can be valuable tools for caregivers seeking to establish a kind and encouraging atmosphere so that their children can flourish. By understanding the unique needs and sensitivities of children and babies and following safety guidelines, caregivers can use aromatherapy's healing properties to encourage the health, happiness, and well-being of their youngest family members.

Aromatherapy for Seniors: Enhancing Quality of Life

Aromatherapy for seniors offers a gentle and holistic approach to enhancing their quality of life by addressing physical, emotional, and cognitive challenges commonly associated with aging. Essential oils, which come from various plants and flowers, contain potent therapeutic properties that can be harnessed to support seniors' overall well-being and promote a sense of comfort, relaxation, and vitality in their golden years. From managing chronic pain and promoting better sleep to alleviating symptoms of anxiety and depression, aromatherapy can play a valuable role in supporting seniors' health and enhancing their quality of life as they age.

One of the primary ways in which aromatherapy can benefit seniors is by managing chronic pain and discomfort. Elderly people frequently suffer from arthritis, muscle stiffness, and joint pain. Lavender, peppermint, and eucalyptus essential oils are among those that have analgesic and anti-inflammatory qualities that can help reduce these symptoms. Massaging these oils into affected areas or adding them to a warm bath can help reduce pain and promote relaxation, providing seniors with natural and effective relief from chronic pain without the side effects of conventional pain medications. Additionally, aromatherapy can help seniors manage neuropathic pain, such as diabetic neuropathy or post-herpetic neuralgia, by soothing nerve endings and promoting better circulation.

Moreover, aromatherapy can benefit seniors by promoting better sleep quality and reducing insomnia. Essential oils with calming qualities, like bergamot, cedarwood, and chamomile, are well-known for promoting sound sleep and calming the body and mind. Seniors can create a peaceful and relaxing environment that promotes sleep by diffusing these oils in their bedroom before bed or by adding a few drops to a warm compress. This will help them sleep better and wake up feeling revitalized. Additionally, by encouraging relaxation and minimizing nocturnal disruptions, aromatherapy can aid in the relief of symptoms connected to restless leg syndrome and other sleep disorders like sleep apnea.

Additionally, aromatherapy helps seniors by easing the symptoms of sadness and anxiety and enhancing emotional well-being. Elderly people frequently face tension, depression, and loneliness. Essential oils with mood-enhancing and uplifting qualities, such lavender, geranium, and ylang-ylang, might help. To help increase the production of neurotransmitters like dopamine and serotonin, which aid regulate mood and promote feelings of contentment and happiness, these oils can be inhaled or applied topically. Additionally, aromatherapy can help seniors cope with significant transitions in life, including retiring or losing a loved one, by providing a safe and natural way to process and express their emotions.

Additionally, aromatherapy supports cognitive function and fosters focus and mental clarity, which is beneficial for seniors. Essential oils with cognitive-enhancing qualities, such lemon, peppermint, and rosemary, are believed to assist seniors' mental alertness, memory, and focus. Diffusing these oils in the home or using them in aromatherapy inhalers can help stimulate brain activity, enhance cognitive function, and promote a sense of mental clarity and sharpness. Additionally, through stimulating neural connections and encouraging neuroplasticity in the brain, aromatherapy can assist elders in managing signs of cognitive decline, such as dementia or Alzheimer's disease.

Furthermore, by strengthening the immune system and lowering the risk of infection and disease, aromatherapy can help elderly. Strong antibacterial and immune-boosting qualities found in essential oils like thyme, eucalyptus, and tea tree can help guard against common illnesses and respiratory conditions. These oils can be diffused throughout the house or used in homemade cleaning solutions to help clean the air, get rid of dangerous germs and viruses, and make it healthier so that senior citizens can live longer. Additionally, incorporating aromatherapy into daily self-care routines can help seniors strengthen their immune systems and improve their resilience to illness and infection.

Furthermore, aromatherapy can benefit seniors by promoting social engagement and fostering a sense of connection and community. Many seniors may experience feelings of isolation and loneliness as they age, especially if they live alone or have limited mobility. Participating in aromatherapy workshops, support groups, or recreational activities can allow seniors to socialize, connect with others, and build meaningful relationships. Additionally, engaging in aromatherapy practices with loved ones or caregivers can strengthen bonds and create opportunities for shared experiences and memories, fostering a sense of belonging and purpose in seniors' lives.

In conclusion, aromatherapy offers a valuable and holistic approach to enhancing seniors' quality of life, supporting their overall well-being, and promoting a sense of comfort, relaxation, and vitality as they age. Seniors can effectively manage chronic pain, enhance cognitive function, boost immunological function, alleviate symptoms of anxiety and depression, improve sleep quality, and promote social engagement and connection by utilizing the medicinal characteristics of essential oils. While aromatherapy should not replace conventional medical treatments or therapies for seniors, it can serve as a valuable complement to existing care, offering seniors additional tools and resources for promoting their health and well-being in their golden years. As research in this area continues to grow, aromatherapy has the potential to play an increasingly important role in supporting seniors' health and enhancing their quality of life as they age.

Aromatherapy for Pets: Supporting Their Health and Well-being

Pets are part of our life and their health and wellbeing are also important for their owners therefore aromatherapy for pets offers a natural and holistic approach to supporting their health and well-being by harnessing the therapeutic properties of essential oils. Similar to the many advantages aromatherapy offers people, it can also be very beneficial to our animal companions, such as horses, dogs, cats, and other animals. Aromatherapy can significantly improve a pet's overall quality of life by fostering relaxation, lowering anxiety, easing discomfort, and bolstering the immune system. But, it's important to use caution when handling essential oils and speak with a veterinarian before adding aromatherapy to your pet's daily regimen.

One of the primary ways aromatherapy can benefit pets is by promoting relaxation and reducing pet's stress and anxiety. Pets can live in a calm and serene atmosphere thanks to the relaxing and soothing qualities of essential oils like bergamot, lavender, and chamomile. These oils can be diffused throughout the house or a pet's bedding to help reduce anxiety and tension, particularly during tense times like thunderstorms, fireworks, or vet appointments. Additionally, aromatherapy can benefit pets who suffer from separation anxiety or fear of travel, helping them feel more calm and secure in unfamiliar environments.

Moreover, aromatherapy can benefit pets by providing natural relief from pain and discomfort. Pets with arthritis symptoms, joint discomfort, and muscular stiffness may find relief with essential oils with analgesic and anti-inflammatory qualities, such as frankincense, ginger, and helichrysum. Pets with chronic pain disorders can benefit from massage treatment or topical application of these oils diluted in a carrier oil to help relieve pain and inflammation, increase mobility, and enhance overall comfort and well-being. Additionally, aromatherapy can be beneficial for pets recovering from surgery or injury, helping to speed up the healing process and reduce the need for conventional pain medications.

Moreover, aromatherapy helps pets by bolstering their immune systems and enhancing their general well-being. Essential oils like eucalyptus and tea tree, and thyme have antimicrobial and immune-boosting properties that can help protect against common infections and illnesses in pets. Diffusing these oils in the home or using homemade cleaning products can help purify the air, get rid of dangerous bacteria and viruses, and make your pet's environment healthier so they can live longer. A pet's immune system can be strengthened and their resistance to disease and infection increased by adding aromatherapy to their daily routine, which will enhance their general health and wellbeing.

In additon, aromatherapy can benefit pets by promoting skin and coat health and reducing symptoms of skin conditions such as itching, inflammation, and allergies. Pets with skin problems can benefit from the calming and anti-inflammatory qualities of essential oils like lavender, chamomile, and geranium, which can also lessen irritation and encourage healing. These oils can be used to improve the general health of the skin and coat of pets by diluting them in a carrier oil and applying it directly to problematic areas, or by mixing them into a shampoo or spray. Aromatherapy also can help pets with seasonal allergies or environmental sensitivities by reducing inflammation and strengthening the skin's natural defenses against allergens.

Furthermore, aromatherapy improves the emotional health of animals and strengthens the link between them and their caregivers. Essential oils such as cedarwood, vetiver, and ylang-ylang are known for their grounding and balancing properties, aiding in the reduction of behavioral problems, tension, and anxiety in pets. Diffusing these oils in the home or massage therapy can help calm nervous pets, promote relaxation, and foster greater trust and connection between pets and their owners. Additionally, aromatherapy can be beneficial for pets experiencing grief or trauma, helping them process and handle challenging emotions in a secure and encouraging setting.

What is more, aromatherapy can benefit pets by promoting respiratory health and reducing symptoms of respiratory conditions such as coughing, wheezing, and congestion. Essential oils having decongestant and expectorant qualities, such eucalyptus, peppermint, and lemon, assist pets with respiratory problems breathe more easily by clearing their nasal passages and reducing inflammation. Diffusing these oils in the home or using them in a steam inhalation treatment can help alleviate symptoms and improve respiratory function, allowing pets to breathe more comfortably and effectively. However, it is essential to use caution when diffusing essential oils around pets, as some oils can be irritating or toxic if ingested or inhaled in large quantities.

In a nutshell, aromatherapy has many positive effects on the physical, emotional, and mental health of pets and provides a holistic, natural approach to promoting their health and well-being. Essential oils can significantly improve the general quality of life for pets by fostering calm, lowering anxiety, relieving pain, and bolstering the immune system. However, before adding essential oils to a pet's daily care regimen, use caution while using aromatherapy and speak with a veterinarian. Pet owners can contribute to the happier, healthier, and more active lives of their furry pets by employing aromatherapy in a responsible and safe manner.

CHAPTER IX

DIY Aromatherapy Recipes and Blends

How to Blend simply at home for Relaxation and Stress Relief

It can be fun and beneficial to use basic essential oil blends for relaxation and stress reduction to support balance and general well-being. Essential oils are made from a variety of herbs and flowers and have strong medicinal qualities that can ease physical and mental stress as well as anxiety. Combining different essential oils in carefully crafted blends can create synergistic effects that enhance their benefits and create a powerful tool for promoting relaxation and stress relief.

One of the most popular essential oils for relaxation and stress relief is lavender. Due to its well-known ability to calm and soothe, lavender oil is a great option for encouraging relaxation and lowering tension and anxiety levels. By diffusing lavender oil throughout the house or using a small amount in a warm bath, you can create a serene and calm environment that promotes relaxation and well-being. Also, lavender oil can be applied topically to pulse points or diluted in a carrier oil for massage to help soothe tense muscles and promote relaxation.

Another essential oil commonly used for relaxation and stress relief is chamomile. Chamomile oil is known for its gentle and calming effects, making it an ideal choice for promoting relaxation and reducing tension and anxiety. Diffusing chamomile oil in the bedroom before bedtime or adding a few drops to a warm compress can help promote restful sleep and reduce nighttime restlessness. In order to help calm irritated skin and encourage relaxation, chamomile oil can also be administered topically after being water down in a carrier oil.

Other essential oils that can be used for relieving stress and relaxation, in addition to lavender and chamomile, include frankincense, ylang-ylang, and bergamot. Because of its uplifting and mood-enhancing qualities, bergamot oil is a great option for encouraging relaxation and lowering stress and anxiety. Because of its well-known balancing and relaxing properties, ylang-ylang oil is a great option for encouraging relaxation and lowering tension and frustration levels. Because of its well-known balancing and centering properties, frankincense oil is a great option for encouraging relaxation and lowering anxiety and feelings of overwhelm.

To create a simple blend for relieving stress and relaxing, add a few drops of your chosen essential oils to a diffuser or mix them with a carrier oil for external use. Experiment with different oil combinations will allow to find the best blend for you and your individual needs. Some popular relaxation and stress relief blends include lavender and chamomile, bergamot and ylang-ylang, and frankincense and lavender. Once your blend is ready, apply it frequently as a part of your self-care regimen to ease tension, encourage relaxation, and improve general wellbeing.

Several more methods can aid in promoting relaxation and lowering tension and anxiety levels in addition to using essential oil blends for stress reduction and relaxation. Practicing deep breathing exercises, engaging in regular physical activity, and practicing mindfulness and meditation are all effective ways to help calm the mind and promote relaxation and well-being. Additionally, making time for self-care activities such as taking a warm bath, enjoying a cup of herbal tea, or spending time in nature can help reduce stress and promote relaxation in our daily lives.

All things considered, basic essential oil mixes for relaxation and stress reduction can be an effective tool for fostering balance and general well-being. Combining different crucial oils in carefully crafted blends can create synergistic effects that enhance their benefits and create a powerful tool for promoting relaxation and stress relief. Essential oil blends can help soothe the body, quiet the mind, and encourage a sense of relaxation and well-being in our daily lives whether they are added to a warm bath, diffused in the air, or applied directly to the skin.

Homemade Skin Care and Beauty Products

Homemade skincare and beauty products offer a natural and sustainable alternative to commercial products, allowing individuals to control what they put on their skin and avoid potentially harmful chemicals and additives. A vast array of skincare and cosmetic products that are efficient, reasonably priced, and customized to meet the demands of specific skin care concerns can be made by utilizing basic, natural materials that are easily found in most kitchens. Homemade skin care products can help nourish, hydrate, and rejuvenate the skin, creating a healthy and beautiful complexion. These products range from facial cleansers and masks to moisturizers and serums.

The absence of harsh chemicals and additives usually found in commercial skin care products is one of the main advantages of making your own skin care products. Many commercial skin care products contain synthetic fragrances, preservatives, and other potentially harmful ingredients that can irritate the skin and contribute to various skin concerns such as acne, dryness, and sensitivity. By making your skincare products at home, you can control the ingredients and ensure that you use only safe and natural ingredients that are gentle and nourishing for the skin.

Moreover, homemade skin care products can be customized to suit individual skin care needs and preferences. Whether you have dry, oily, sensitive, or combination skin, homemade recipes are available to address specific skin concerns and achieve desired results. For instance, moisturizing components like avocado oil, shea butter, and coconut oil may be beneficial for dry skin. On the other hand, people with oily or acne-prone skin could favor non-comedogenic, milder ingredients like witch hazel, aloe vera, or jojoba oil. You can create personalized skin care products that meet your unique skin care needs by experimenting with different ingredients and formulations.

Additionally, homemade skin care products are often more affordable than their commercial counterparts, as they require fewer ingredients and do not involve the costs associated with packaging, marketing, and distribution. Fruits, vegetables, herbs, and oils are just a few of the commonly available and reasonably priced bulk items that may be found in health food stores or grocery stores, and are frequently utilized in homemade skin care products. Making your skincare products at home can save money while reducing waste and minimizing your environmental footprint.

Furthermore, homemade skin care products can be more sustainable and eco-friendly than commercial products, as they often involve minimal packaging and make use of environmentally friendly, natural, biodegradable ingredients. Numerous skin care products sold in stores are packaged in plastic tubes or containers, which adds to pollution and damage to the environment. You may lessen your environmental effect and dependency on single-use plastics by manufacturing your skincare items at home.

Depending on your tastes and needs for skin care, you can create a wide variety of homemade skin care products at home. Some popular homemade skin care products include facial cleansers, toners, masks, serums, and moisturizers. Gentle, natural ingredients like oats, yogurt, and honey can be used to make facial cleansers that effectively cleanse the skin without removing its natural oils. Toners can be made using witch hazel, apple cider vinegar, or rose water, which help balance the skin's pH levels and tighten pores. Clay, avocado, and honey are a few substances that can be used to make masks that target particular skin conditions while also nourishing and revitalizing the skin. Serums can be made using vitamin C, hyaluronic acid, or rosehip oil, which help hydrate, brighten, and protect the skin from environmental damage. Moisturizers can be made using shea butter, cocoa butter, or almond oil, which helps hydrate and provide vital minerals and antioxidants to soothe the skin.

Summing up the main points, homemade skincare and beauty products offer a natural, affordable, and sustainable alternative to commercial products, allowing individuals to take control of their skincare routine and avoid potentially harmful chemicals and additives. While using simple, natural ingredients readily available in most kitchens makes it possible to create a large selection of customized, eco-friendly, and efficacious skincare and cosmetic items that are personalized and environmentally friendly. Whether you have dry, oily, sensitive, or combination skin, homemade recipes are available to address specific skin concerns and achieve desired results. By making your skin care products at home, you can nourish, hydrate, and rejuvenate your skin while minimizing your environmental footprint and promoting a healthier, more sustainable lifestyle.

Natural Cleaning Solutions with Essential Oils

Essential oil-based natural cleaning solutions are a secure, efficient, and green substitute for traditional cleaning products, which are frequently loaded with toxic chemicals. By harnessing critical oils' natural antibacterial, antiviral, and antifungal properties, it is possible to create homemade cleaning solutions that effectively clean and disinfect surfaces while promoting a healthier indoor environment for humans and pets. From countertops and floors to bathrooms and kitchens, essential oils can tackle many cleaning tasks, leaving behind a fresh, uplifting scent without synthetic fragrances or harsh chemicals.

The strong antibacterial qualities of essential oils are one of the main advantages of utilizing them for cleaning. Strong disinfectants for use in cleaning solutions are present in a variety of essential oils, such as tea tree, lemon, and eucalyptus. These oils contain chemicals that have been demonstrated to efficiently kill bacteria, viruses, and fungi. For example, tea tree oil is known for its broad-spectrum antimicrobial activity, making it an excellent choice for disinfecting surfaces in the home. Lemon oil is a common ingredient in DIY cleaning solutions since it is also very good at eliminating bacteria and germs.

Moreover, essential oils are natural deodorizers, helping to eliminate smells and leave a clean, fresh aroma in their wake. Unlike synthetic fragrances in many commercial cleaning products, essential oils provide an honest and uplifting aroma that might enhance the quality of the air indoors and create a more pleasant environment for occupants. Popular essential oils for deodorizing and freshening the air include lavender, peppermint, and orange, which smell delightful and have natural antibacterial properties that help eliminate odors at their source.

Additionally, essential oils are non-toxic and biodegradable, making them safer for children, pets, and the environment than conventional cleaning products. Bleach and other harsh chemicals are used in a lot of professional cleaning products, ammonia, and phthalates, which can be harmful if ingested or inhaled and can contribute to indoor air pollution and environmental degradation. Using natural cleaning solutions with essential oils can reduce exposure to potentially harmful chemicals and create a safer, healthier living environment for your family and the planet.

Moreover, essential oils are adaptable and can be employed in a variety of household cleaning applications. For example, tea tree oil can be added to homemade all-purpose cleaners to disinfect countertops, sinks, and other surfaces. Lemon oil can be added to floor cleaners to cut through grease and grime and leave a fresh citrus scent behind. Peppermint oil can be added to bathroom cleaners to kill germs and bacteria and restore a cooling, refreshing aroma. With a few simple ingredients and some basic knowledge of essential oils, you can create a wide range of effective cleaning solutions that are safe, affordable, and eco-friendly.

Gather essential ingredients such as distilled water, white vinegar, baking soda, and liquid castile soap to make your natural cleaning solutions with essential oils. Then, please choose your favorite essential oils based on their cleaning properties and aroma preferences. Tea tree, lemon, and lavender are excellent choices for general cleaning, while peppermint and eucalyptus are perfect for freshening the air and eliminating odors. Experiment with different combinations of oils and adjust the ratios to suit your personal preferences and cleaning needs.

One popular homemade cleaning solution is an all-purpose cleaner with vinegar, water, and essential oils. Combine distilled water and white vinegar in a spray bottle, and add several drops of essential oils. Shake well before each use and spray onto surfaces such as countertops, sinks, and appliances. Enjoy the fresh, clean aroma of your homemade cleaning solution as you wipe it clean with a damp cloth or sponge.

To sum up, natural cleaning solutions using essential oils present a secure, efficient, and sustainable substitute for traditional cleaning agents. Making use of essential oils' inherent antibacterial, deodorizing, and uplifting qualities, one can make DIY cleaning solutions that not only efficiently clean and disinfect surfaces but also foster a healthier indoor atmosphere for both people and dogs. Whether you're cleaning countertops, floors, bathrooms, or kitchens, essential oils can tackle many cleaning tasks, leaving behind a fresh, uplifting scent without the need for synthetic fragrances or harsh chemicals. Making your natural cleaning solutions with essential oils can reduce exposure to potentially harmful chemicals, create a safer, healthier living environment, and contribute to a more sustainable planet.

CHAPTER X

Aromatherapy Ethics and Safety

Understanding Dilution and Dosage Guidelines

It's critical to comprehend dose and dilution recommendations when employing essential oils in aromatherapy and other applications to ensure safety and effectiveness. Dilution refers to mixing essential oils with a carrier oil or different base to reduce their concentration and minimize the risk of skin irritation or sensitivity. Dosage, on the other hand, refers to the amount of essential oil used in a specific application, whether for topical use, inhalation, or internal consumption. People can optimize the advantages of essential oils while lowering the possibility of negative reactions or side effects by adhering to the recommended dilution and dose standards.

Realizing that essential oils are extremely concentrated compounds that can result in skin irritation, allergic responses, or other negative effects if used undiluted or in excessive quantities is one of the most important parts of comprehending dilution and dosing standards. The strong aromatic chemicals found in essential oils, which are produced from a variety of plant components including leaves, flowers, bark, and roots, are what give them their medicinal qualities. But these substances can also cause skin irritation, especially when applied topically or to delicate body parts.

Diluting essential oils safely for topical use is recommended when using a carrier oil, such as jojoba, coconut, almond, or grapeseed oil. Carriers reduce the likelihood of sensitivity or pain in addition to serving as a barrier to shield the skin and dilute essential oils. The recommended dilution ratio for topical use varies depending on the age, skin sensitivity, and health status of the individual, as well as the specific essential oil being used. As a general guideline, a 1-3% dilution ratio is typically recommended for adults, with lower dilution ratios (0.5-1%) for children, elderly individuals, or those with sensitive skin.

When determining the appropriate dosage of essential oils for topical use, it's important to consider factors such as the application's intended purpose, the area of the body being treated, and the individual's age, weight, and overall health. There are some essential oils that are more potent and may require lower dosages, while others may be used more liberally depending on the desired effect. It's also important to consider the cumulative effect of repeated applications over time, as prolonged or excessive use of specific essential oils can lead to sensitization or other adverse reactions.

In addition to topical use, essential oils can be inhaled through diffusion, steam inhalation, or direct inhalation from a bottle or tissue. Inhalation is a popular method for experiencing the aromatic benefits of essential oils, which can help promote relaxation, improve mood, and support respiratory health. When using essential oils for inhalation, it's important to consider factors such as the individual's sensitivity to intense aromas, the duration and frequency of exposure, and any pre-existing respiratory conditions or allergies.

Dosage guidelines for inhalation can vary depending on the method of administration and the specific essential oil being used. For instance, it's usually okay to use 5–10 essential oil drops for every 100 milliliters of water in a diffuser when distributing them across a space. However, the exact dosage may vary depending on the room's size and the aroma's desired strength. Similarly, when using essential oils for steam inhalation, it's important to use caution and start with a low dosage to avoid overwhelming the senses or causing irritation to the respiratory tract.

It can be also added additionally to topical and inhalation, some essential oils which may be used internally for their therapeutic benefits. However, this should be done under the guidance of a qualified healthcare professional. Internal use of essential oils typically involves diluting the oil in a carrier oil or adding it to food or beverages, such as herbal teas or smoothies. Dosage guidelines for internal use are highly variable. They should be tailored to the individual's specific health needs and the potency and safety profile of the essential oil being used.

To use essential oils in aromatherapy and other applications safely and successfully, one must be aware of dose and dilution recommendations. People can reduce the possibility of negative reactions or side effects while optimizing the therapeutic advantages of these strong plant extracts by correctly diluting essential oils and adhering to suggested dosage guidelines. Whether used topically, for inhalation, or internally, essential oils can promote health, wellness, and vitality when used responsibly and by established safety guidelines.

Safety Precautions and Contraindications

Safety precautions and understanding contraindications are paramount when using essential oils and aromatherapy to ensure the well-being and health of individuals. Essential oils are powerful compounds that need to be handled and used carefully because of their concentrated nature and potential for negative reactions, even if they have many medicinal benefits. Practitioners can reduce hazards and encourage the safe and efficient use of essential oils in a variety of applications by following safety protocols and being aware of contraindications.

One of the fundamental safety precautions when using essential oils is to always dilute them properly before applying them to the skin. Undiluted essential oils can cause skin irritation, sensitization, or even burns, especially in individuals with sensitive skin or allergies. Essential oils can be made less potent and less likely to cause negative reactions by diluting them with a carrier oil. The recommended dilution ratio varies depending on factors such as the individual's age, skin sensitivity, and the specific essential oil being used, but as a general guideline, a dilution ratio of 1-3% is typically recommended for adults, with lower dilution ratios (0.5-1%) for children, elderly individuals, or those with sensitive skin.

Make sure an essential oil is appropriately diluted and patch tested before using it topically, especially if you have sensitive skin or are prone to allergies. A patch test involves applying a tiny amount of diluted essential oil to a small area of skin, such as the inner forearm, and waiting 24 to 48 hours to see whether there are any adverse effects. If redness, itching, or irritation occurs, it's best to avoid using the essential oil or diluting it further before using it again.

Being aware of phototoxic essential oils, which can burn or irritate skin when exposed to sunshine or UV radiation, is another crucial safety precaution. Furanocoumarins are substances found in phototoxic essential oils that increase skin sensitivity to sunlight and may cause phytophotodermatitis. Common phototoxic essential oils include citrus oils such as bergamot, lemon, lime, grapefruit and certain herbs like angelica, fennel, and rue. To avoid phototoxic reactions, it's best to avoid applying phototoxic essential oils to the skin before going out in the sun or using them in goods that are going to be in direct sunlight, such as body oils or lotions.

Additionally, certain essential oils may have specific contraindications or precautions based on individual health conditions or medications. For example, individuals with epilepsy or seizure disorders should use caution when using stimulating essential oils such as rosemary, sage, or eucalyptus, as they may trigger seizures in susceptible individuals. Additionally, women who are expecting should use essential oils with caution, especially in the first trimester, as some of them may stimulate the uterus or pose other hazards to the growing fetus. Before using essential oils while pregnant, it is imperative to see a qualified healthcare professional, particularly if you have any underlying medical conditions.

Moreover, essential oils should only be taken under the supervision of a licensed healthcare provider because consuming too much of some oils could render them dangerous or toxic. While some essential oils may be safe for internal use in small quantities and under the supervision of a trained practitioner, others may cause gastrointestinal upset, liver toxicity, or other adverse effects. When taking essential oils internally, it's important to proceed with caution, adhere to dosage recommendations, and always select pure, high-quality essential oils that are safe for internal use.

In addition to topical and internal use, essential oils can be inhaled through diffusion, steam inhalation, or direct inhalation from a bottle or tissue. While inhalation is generally considered safe for most individuals, it's important to use caution when diffusing essential oils in enclosed spaces or around individuals with respiratory conditions or sensitivities to intense aromas. Some essential oils may trigger respiratory symptoms or exacerbate existing conditions, so choosing well-tolerated oils and avoiding prolonged or excessive inhalation is necessary.

All things considered, safety precautions and understanding contraindications are essential when using essential oils and aromatherapy to ensure the well-being and health of individuals. By following proper dilution guidelines, performing patch tests, and being mindful of phototoxicity and individual contraindications, practitioners can minimize the risk of adverse reactions and promote the safe and effective use of essential oils in various applications. Before using essential oils, it's also crucial to speak with a licensed healthcare provider, particularly if you have any underlying medical conditions, are pregnant, or are on medication. With proper safety precautions and knowledge, essential oils can be valuable tools for promoting health, wellness, and vitality.

Ethical Sourcing and Sustainability in Aromatherapy

Ethical sourcing and sustainability are increasingly important to consider in aromatherapy as the demand for essential oils and concerns about environmental impact and social responsibility grow. Ethical sourcing refers to the practices and principles involved in obtaining crucial oils in a fair, transparent manner that respects both people and the planet. On the other hand, sustainability focuses on ensuring that essential oil production and harvesting methods are environmentally responsible and do not deplete natural resources or harm ecosystems. By prioritizing ethical sourcing and sustainability, aromatherapy practitioners can support the well-being of communities, protect biodiversity, and promote the long-term viability of the aromatherapy industry.

One of the fundamental principles of ethical sourcing is transparency in the supply chain, which involves tracing the journey of essential oils from cultivation and harvesting to processing and distribution. Transparency helps ensure that essential oils are sourced from reputable suppliers who adhere to fair labor practices, environmental regulations, and quality standards. It also allows consumers to make informed choices about their products and supports companies prioritizing ethical sourcing and sustainability.

Fairtrade certification is one way to promote ethical sourcing in the aromatherapy industry by ensuring that producers receive fair wages and working conditions for their labor. Appropriate trade organizations work to empower small-scale farmers and producers, particularly in developing countries, by providing access to markets, fair prices, and support for sustainable farming practices. By purchasing honest trade-certified essential oils, consumers can support the livelihoods of farmers and workers and contribute to poverty alleviation and community development initiatives.

Another aspect of ethical sourcing is respecting indigenous knowledge and cultural heritage associated with producing essential oils. Many essential oils come from plants that indigenous communities have used for centuries for their medicinal, aromatic, and spiritual properties. It is necessary to recognize and honor indigenous peoples' traditional knowledge and practices and ensure they are compensated and involved in essential oil production and trade decision-making processes.

Sustainability is another critical consideration in aromatherapy, as the demand for essential oils can pressure ecosystems and biodiversity if not managed responsibly. Sustainable harvesting practices aim to minimize the environmental impact of actual oil production by ensuring that plants are harvested in a way that allows them to regenerate and thrive over time. This may involve techniques such as selective harvesting, where only a portion of the plant material is collected, leaving the rest to continue growing and reproducing.

In addition to sustainable harvesting, efforts to promote biodiversity conservation and habitat protection are essential for the long-term sustainability of actual oil production. In order to keep ecosystems robust and plant populations resilient in the face of environmental problems like habitat degradation and climate change, biodiversity is essential. The aromatherapy industry can contribute to biodiversity conservation and ecosystem restoration efforts by protecting natural habitats and supporting agroforestry and reforestation initiatives.

Furthermore, sustainable agriculture practices, such as organic and regenerative agriculture, play a vital role in ensuring the sustainability of essential oil production. Organic certification prohibits synthetic pesticides, fertilizers, and genetically modified organisms (GMOs), helping to protect soil health, water quality, and biodiversity. Regenerative agriculture goes a step further by rebuilding soil health, enhancing ecosystem services, and promoting carbon sequestration to lessen the impacts of climate change.

Certification programs such as organic and sustainable agriculture assure consumers that essential oils are produced using environmentally friendly and socially responsible practices. These accreditations assist customers in making wise decisions and encourage businesses that place a high priority on sustainability and ethical sourcing. Certifications like FairWild and Fair For Life, in addition to organic and sustainable agriculture certifications, concentrate particularly on fair trade and social responsibility in the wild collection and cultivation of botanical ingredients.

Summing up the main points such as ethical sourcing and sustainability are essential principles in aromatherapy that promote fair labor practices, environmental stewardship, and the industry's long-term viability. By prioritizing transparency, fair trade, indigenous rights, biodiversity conservation, and sustainable agriculture, aromatherapy practitioners can support the well-being of communities, protect ecosystems, and ensure that essential oils are produced and traded in an ethical, responsible, and environmentally sustainable manner. Through collaboration, education, and advocacy, the aromatherapy industry can continue to evolve toward a more honest and sustainable future that benefits people, plants, and the planet.

CHAPTER XI

The Future of Aromatherapy

Emerging Trends and Innovations in Aromatherapy

Emerging trends and innovations in aromatherapy are shaping the future of this ancient healing practice, offering new opportunities for wellness, personal care, and holistic health. As our understanding of the therapeutic properties of essential oils deepens and technology advances, aromatherapy continues to evolve, with new applications, products, and techniques emerging to meet the needs of modern consumers. From personalized aromatherapy solutions to high-tech delivery systems, these innovations are driving the growth and popularity of aromatherapy in diverse fields such as healthcare, beauty, hospitality, and beyond.

One of the most significant trends in aromatherapy is the growing interest in personalized solutions tailored to individual needs and preferences. Personalized aromatherapy considers a person's unique scent preferences, health concerns, and lifestyle choices to create customized blends and treatments that address specific wellness goals. This approach allows for greater flexibility and effectiveness in using essential oils to support physical, emotional, and mental well-being, catering to the diverse needs of today's consumers.

Advancements in technology have also led to innovations in aromatherapy delivery systems, making it easier and more convenient to enjoy the benefits of essential oils anytime, anywhere. Aromatherapy diffusers, for example, have become increasingly sophisticated, with features such as adjustable intensity settings, programmable timers, and wireless connectivity, allowing users to create personalized scent experiences at home or on the go. Portable diffusers and inhalers are also gaining popularity, offering discreet and convenient ways to enjoy the aromatic benefits of essential oils throughout the day.

In addition to traditional diffusion methods, new technologies such as microencapsulation and nanotechnology are being explored to enhance the delivery and efficacy of essential oils in topical and internal applications. Microencapsulation involves encapsulating critical oil molecules in microscopic spheres or particles, which can be incorporated into products such as skincare formulations, supplements, and functional foods. This technology helps to protect the volatile compounds in essential oils from degradation and oxidation, ensuring maximum potency and stability over time.

On the other hand, nanotechnology involves manipulating nanoscale materials to enhance their properties and interactions with biological systems. In aromatherapy, nanotechnology is used to create nanoemulsions and nanostructured delivery systems that improve essential oils' solubility, absorption, and bioavailability in topical and internal applications. These advanced delivery systems allow for more targeted and efficient delivery of important oil compounds to the body, enhancing their therapeutic effects and reducing the risk of adverse reactions.

Another emerging trend in aromatherapy is the integration of aromatherapy with other complementary and alternative therapies to create synergistic treatment approaches that address the whole person. For example, aromatherapy massage combines essential oils' therapeutic benefits with massage therapy's healing touch to promote relaxation, reduce stress, and alleviate muscular tension. Similarly, aromatherapy yoga combines the inhalation of essential oils with yoga practice to enhance mindfulness, deepen relaxation, and support emotional balance.

Furthermore, aromatherapy is increasingly being used in clinical settings as an adjunctive therapy to conventional medical treatments, particularly in areas such as pain management, mental health, and supportive care for chronic conditions. Research studies have demonstrated the efficacy of aromatherapy in reducing pain, anxiety, and depression, boosting the general quality of life and quality of sleep for people with a range of medical issues. As evidence of the therapeutic benefits of aromatherapy continues to accumulate, its integration into mainstream healthcare is expected to grow, providing new opportunities for collaboration between aromatherapists, healthcare providers, and researchers.

In the realm of beauty and personal care, aromatherapy is also experiencing a renaissance, with natural and organic skincare brands incorporating essential oils into their formulations to enhance their products' sensory experience and therapeutic benefits. From aromatherapy-infused facial oils and serums to botanical perfumes and bath products, consumers are increasingly seeking natural and holistic alternatives to conventional skincare products that promote health and well-being from the inside out.

As can be seen, emerging trends and innovations in aromatherapy are transforming how we approach health, wellness, and self-care, offering new opportunities for personalized, holistic, and integrative approaches to healing. From personalized aromatherapy solutions and high-tech delivery systems to integrating aromatherapy with other complementary therapies and its use in clinical settings, aromatherapy encourages change and adaptation to satisfy the demands of contemporary consumers. As research into the therapeutic benefits of essential oils continues to expand and technology advances, the future of aromatherapy looks brighter than ever, with new possibilities for promoting health, happiness, and harmony for individuals and communities worldwide.

Aromatherapy Research and Scientific Advancements

Aromatherapy research and scientific advancements have been crucial in elevating aromatherapy from a traditional healing practice to a respected and evidence-based modality in modern healthcare. Over the past few decades, there has been a significant increase in research studies. They were investigating the therapeutic properties, mechanisms of action, and clinical applications of essential oils, resulting in an expanding corpus of scientific data proving their safety and effectiveness. From laboratory studies elucidating the biochemical pathways of essential oil compounds to clinical trials evaluating their therapeutic effects in humans, aromatherapy research has made significant strides in advancing our understanding of essential oils' potential benefits and applications for health and well- being.

One area of aromatherapy research that has seen significant growth is the study of the pharmacological properties of essential oils and their chemical constituents. Essential oils are intricate blends of volatile plant-based chemicals, each having a distinct chemical makeup and medicinal use. A lot of research has been done to find out what the bioactive chemicals in essential oils are, how they work, and what effects they have on the body, such as their ability to kill bacteria, reduce inflammation, ease pain, calm people down, and make them feel less anxious. The mechanisms of action of essential oils and their potential uses in the prevention and treatment of many medical diseases have been better understood thanks to these studies.

In addition to laboratory research, clinical trials have been conducted to evaluate the efficacy of aromatherapy interventions in diverse populations and settings. Clinical studies have explored the use of aromatherapy for pain management, stress reduction, sleep improvement, mood enhancement, and supportive care for chronic diseases such as cancer, fibromyalgia, and dementia. While many clinical trials have reported positive outcomes and benefits associated with aromatherapy interventions, further research is needed to establish the optimal protocols, dosages, and delivery methods for specific health conditions and populations.

One of the challenges in aromatherapy research is the variability and complexity of essential oils, which can affect their therapeutic efficacy and reproducibility. Plant species, growing conditions, harvesting procedures, extraction methods, and storage conditions can all have an impact on the chemical make-up and biological activity of essential oils. Measures for quality control and standardization are crucial to ensure the consistency and reliability of critical oil products used in research studies and clinical practice. Researchers can now accurately study and characterize the chemical makeup of essential oils and find trace compounds that may help them work as medicines thanks to improvements in analytical techniques like gas chromatography-mass spectrometry (GC-MS) and nuclear magnetic resonance (NMR) spectroscopy.

There is another area of aromatherapy research that has gained attention in recent years. It is the investigation of the mechanisms of action underlying the effects of essential oils on the body and mind. Studies have shown that essential oils can exert their therapeutic effects through various mechanisms, including modulation of neurotransmitter levels, regulation of inflammatory pathways, modulation of autonomic nervous system activity, and modulation of gene expression. By elucidating the molecular mechanisms by which essential oils interact with biological systems, researchers can better understand their therapeutic potential and identify new targets for drug development and therapy.

Furthermore, researchers are now able to examine how aromatherapy affects brain activity and function thanks to developments in neuroimaging methods like positron emission tomography (PET) and functional magnetic resonance imaging (fMRI). Neuroimaging studies have shown that inhaling certain essential oils can modulate brain regions involved in emotion, memory, and stress response, leading to mood, cognition, and behavior changes. The use of aromatherapy as a non-pharmacological remedy for mental diseases, such as anxiety, depression, and post-traumatic stress disorder (PTSD), has scientific backing thanks to these discoveries.

In addition, research into the safety and toxicity of essential oils has also been a focus of aromatherapy inquiry. While essential oils are thought to be safe when used according to instructions, some people may react negatively to them, especially if they use large amounts or apply them to sensitive areas of their skin. Toxicological studies have evaluated essential oils' acute and chronic toxicity in animal models and human subjects to assess their safety profile and identify potential risks associated with long-term or excessive use. Additionally, pharmacokinetic studies have investigated the absorption, distribution, metabolism, and excretion of essential oil compounds in the body to understand their pharmacokinetic properties better and optimize their therapeutic use.

To sum this up, aromatherapy research and scientific advancements have contributed significantly to our understanding of essential oils' therapeutic potential and mechanisms of action. From lab studies that explain the pharmacological properties of essential oil compounds to clinical trials that test how well they work in different settings and populations, aromatherapy research has taught us a lot about the health and wellness benefits and uses of essential oils. Continued investment in research and collaboration between scientists, healthcare professionals, and aromatherapists is essential to advance our knowledge of aromatherapy further and unlock its full potential as a safe, effective, and evidence- based healing modality.

Aromatherapy's   Role in Sustainable and Holistic Health Practices

Aromatherapy's role in sustainable and holistic health practices worldwide extends beyond individual well-being to encompass broader environmental sustainability, social responsibility, cultural preservation, and global health equity considerations. Rooted in ancient healing traditions and indigenous knowledge systems, aromatherapy has emerged as a versatile and accessible modality that integrates the therapeutic use of essential oils with principles of sustainability, holistic wellness, and cultural diversity. From traditional healing practices passed down through generations to modern healthcare settings and global wellness industries, aromatherapy's influence on sustainable and holistic health practices is diverse and far-reaching, encompassing various applications and approaches across different cultures, communities, and contexts.

One of the critical aspects of aromatherapy's role in sustainable and holistic health practices worldwide is its emphasis on using natural and renewable resources derived from plants. Essential oils are the primary therapeutic agents used in aromatherapy, which are extracted from various plant parts, including flowers, leaves, stems, bark, and roots, through steam distillation, cold pressing, and solvent extraction. Aromatherapy practitioners can promote health and well-being while supporting the conservation of biodiversity, ecological balance, and sustainable land use practices by harnessing the healing power of nature's botanical treasures. Moreover, cultivating and harvesting aromatic plants for essential oil production can provide economic opportunities for local communities, particularly in rural and indigenous areas where plant-based industries play a vital role in livelihoods and cultural heritage preservation.

In addition to promoting environmental sustainability, aromatherapy contributes to holistic health and wellness by addressing physical, emotional, mental, and spiritual aspects of well-being. Essential oils contain bioactive compounds that exert pharmacological effects on the body and mind, influencing physiological processes such as circulation, digestion, respiration, and immune function. Through a variety of applications, such as topical application, inhalation, and massage treatment, numerous illnesses can be treated using aromatherapy, including inflammation, stress, anxiety, depression, sleeplessness, and digestive disorders. Moreover, aromatherapy's holistic approach to health recognizes the interconnectedness between mind, body, and spirit, acknowledging that emotional and spiritual well-being are essential to overall health and vitality.

Furthermore, aromatherapy's role in sustainable and holistic health practices is closely intertwined with cultural diversity, heritage preservation, and community resilience. Many cultures worldwide have long-standing traditions of using aromatic plants and essential oils for healing, spiritual rituals, and cultural ceremonies. Indigenous peoples and traditional healers have deep knowledge of local plant species, their medicinal properties, and sustainable harvesting practices, passed down through oral traditions and experiential learning. By honoring and respecting traditional knowledge systems, aromatherapy practitioners can gain valuable insights into the therapeutic uses of aromatic plants and their cultural significance while promoting cultural diversity, preservation of heritage, and intercultural exchange.

Moreover, aromatherapy's role in sustainable and holistic health practices extends to global health equity and social justice, addressing disparities in access to healthcare, resources, and opportunities. In many parts of the world, particularly in low-income and marginalized communities, access to conventional healthcare services and pharmaceutical drugs may be limited or unaffordable. Aromatherapy offers a cost-effective, accessible, and culturally relevant alternative to traditional medicine, empowering individuals and communities to take control of their health and well-being through natural and holistic approaches. By promoting health literacy, self-care practices, and community empowerment, aromatherapy can help bridge the gap between traditional and modern healthcare systems, foster health equity, and promote social justice in diverse cultural contexts.

Furthermore, aromatherapy's role in sustainable and holistic health practices is increasingly recognized and integrated into mainstream healthcare systems, public health initiatives, and global wellness industries. In many countries, aromatherapy is used in hospitals, clinics, hospices, and other healthcare settings as an adjunctive therapy to conventional medical treatments, particularly in pain management, stress reduction, supportive care, and palliative care. Aromatherapy is also gaining popularity in spa resorts, wellness retreats, yoga studios, and beauty salons as a complementary therapy for relaxation, rejuvenation, and holistic self-care. In addition, the expanding global wellness market's need for natural and organic products has given educators, practitioners, and business owners new ways to reach a wider audience with their expertise and goods.

Taking everyting said into account, aromatherapy's role in sustainable and holistic health practices worldwide encompasses various applications, approaches, and contexts that promote individual well-being, environmental sustainability, cultural diversity, and global health equity. By harnessing the healing power of nature's botanical treasures, aromatherapy practitioners can support physical, emotional, mental, and spiritual health while fostering greater harmony and balance within ourselves, our communities, and the world around us. As aromatherapy continues to evolve and adapt to adjust to the shifting demands and difficulties of the modern world, its potential to promote sustainable and holistic health practices worldwide remains as vast and diverse as the aromatic plants from which it derives.

CONCLUSION

"Aromas of Wellness: Harnessing Nature's Essence for Health and Harmony" encapsulates the journey into the transformative power of aromatherapy, offering readers a comprehensive exploration of its myriad benefits for physical, emotional, and spiritual well-being. Throughout this book, we have delved into aromatherapy's rich history and origins, traced its evolution from ancient healing traditions to modern healthcare practices, and explored its diverse applications in promoting holistic health and sustainability worldwide.

As we conclude our aromatic odyssey, it becomes evident that the essence of wellness lies in the harmonious integration of mind, body, and spirit. Aromatherapy serves as a bridge between the natural world and our inner landscape, inviting us to reconnect with the healing wisdom of nature and awaken our innate capacity for self-healing and transformation. From the soothing scent of lavender to the refreshing aroma of peppermint, each essential oil offers a unique bouquet of therapeutic benefits, nurturing our physical vitality, soothing our emotional wounds, and uplifting our spirits.

Moreover, "Aromas of Wellness" emphasizes the importance of ethical sourcing, sustainability, and cultural diversity in aromatherapy practices. By honoring the sacred relationship between plants and people, we can cultivate a deeper appreciation for the interconnectedness of all life forms and foster tremendous respect for the natural world. We can guarantee these fragrant gems will be available for centuries to come by practicing fair trade, conscientious cultivation, and responsible harvesting. This will also help to preserve biodiversity, assist local communities, and encourage environmental stewardship.

In essence, "Aromas of Wellness" is more than just a book—it is a testament to the profound potential of aromatherapy to enrich our lives and cultivate a more profound sense of harmony and balance. As we incorporate the principles and practices of aromatherapy into our daily lives, we embark on a journey of self- discovery, healing, and empowerment, guided by the wisdom of nature and the transformative power of scent.

May this book serve as a source of inspiration, guidance, and empowerment for all who seek to harness the healing essence of nature and cultivate a life of wellness and harmony. Let's keep exploring, growing, and learning on our aromatic journey, embracing the gifts of the earth with gratitude and reverence, and weaving the threads of health, happiness, and harmony into the fabric of our lives and our world.

Finally, arotheramy oils can create the scents of well-being and fill our days with happiness, energy, and calm. Moreover they can remind us of the healing potential and beauty of the natural world around us. Let us savor the scents of nature, embrace the wisdom of ancient traditions, and walk the path of wellness with grace and gratitude. For instance the fragrance of flowers and the essence of essential oils, we discover the timeless truth that health and harmony are the birthright of all beings and that by harnessing nature's essence, we can truly thrive in body, mind, and spirit.

Thank you for buying and reading/ listening to our book. If you found this book useful/ helpful please take a few minutes and leave a review on the platform where you purchased our book. Your feedback matters greatly to us.